DEEPENING YOUR PRACTICE

AN ESSENTIAL GUIDE FOR YOGA STUDENTS AND TEACHERS

By: Ryan Glidden

Published by: MOSAIC Institute For Human Development LLC

811 25th Street Suite 102, San Diego CA 92102

www.exploremosaic.com

Printed in the United States of America by lulu publishing www.lulu.com

First Printing, 2019

ISBN 978-0-359-36054-3

Deepening Your Practice reflects the views and personal experiences of the author. this book is intended to complement, not replace, professional medical advice, diagnosis and treatment. If you have or suspect you have a medical problem, immediately see your doctor or a professional health-care provider. No medical claims are made as to effects or outcomes of the exercises described in this book.

Edited by: Thalia Suzuma

Cover Photography: Meredith Coe

Interior Photography: Elizabeth Cavagnaro

Interior illustrations both created by Ryan Glidden and purchased from Vectorstock, www.vectorstock.com

Table of Contents

"Yoga is the rule book for playing the game of Life, but in this game no one needs to lose. It is tough, and you need to train hard. It requires the willingness to think for yourself, to observe and correct, and to surmount occasional setbacks. It demands honesty, sustained application, and above all love in your heart. If you are interested to understand what it means to be a human being, placed between earth and sky, if you are interested in where you come from and where you will be able to go, if you want happiness and long for freedom, then you have already begun to take the first steps toward the journey inward.

The rules of nature cannot be bent. They are impersonal and implacable. But we do play with them. By accepting nature's challenge and joining the game, we find ourselves on a windswept and exciting journey that will pay benefits commensurate to the time and effort we put in- the lowest being our ability to tie our own shoelaces when we are eighty and the highest being the opportunity to taste the essence of life itself."

- Light on Life, by BKS Iyengar

PREFACE

There I was. Sitting on a yoga mat in a room that must have been 115°. Ok. . . This room is hot, I thought to myself. And the humidity! It was already hard to breathe, and we hadn't even started yet.

Days before, Melissa Love, the girl who worked in the regional office of our company, the one who all the guys in the yard wanted to take a shot at dating, had suggested I come to yoga with her. I had heard of yoga but had never practiced before.

Well, I thought, if it means we can go out on another date, I'm in. How hard could it really be? I had grown up playing football in New England summers and winters from the time I was ten all the way through college. It couldn't be worse than triple session practices in full pads in the middle of August. I was wrong!

I was halfway through the 26-pose sequence when I started to see little flashes of light. Like tiny stars sporadically bursting into existence and then fading away. The last time that had happened was when I had been hit in the head by an oversized linebacker in college.

When that passed, the instructor seemed to be at the opposite end of a tunnel. His voice sounded like it was 50 yards away.

"Ok. . . I'm going to pass out," I thought.

I took a deep breath and looked down and over to my right. A rather large woman was moving through the poses like a kid dancing. She had such ease and grace and there seemed to be no struggle whatsoever.

"That's it," I told myself. "If this woman, who I must be in better shape than, does not leave this room, I am not going to leave this room. They will have to carry me out of here unconscious."

I'd say at times I probably wasn't too far away from this being the case, but I made it. Soaked through to the bone I reached Savasana, the final resting posture. I learned later it was called corpse pose. That seems about right, I thought. I felt like I'd almost died.

After dragging myself into the locker room, gathering my wits and getting dressed, I met Melissa outside.

"What did you think?" she asked.

"It was great," I lied. The class was one of the hardest things I had ever done.

But in fact I had never felt so relaxed in my body. I was intrigued. This was a new physical challenge and I wanted to master it, and I was also enjoying this feeling of compete relaxation now that the class was over. I admit, for a while, I was scared to go back to that class, but I was intrigued by this "yoga" thing, and I found a vinyasa studio closer to where I lived. I had been told that vinyasa yoga was easier for beginners than hot yoga.

My first class at the vinyasa studio was not nearly as intense – the room was at a normal temperature – but again I found new sensations in my body that I never expected.

I had spent years of my life powerlifting, gaining weight and muscle. I could push press 200lbs above my head but here I was, in Downward Facing Dog pose for no more than 30 seconds, and my arms were shaking like leaves in the wind. I thought my shoulders were going to give.

I enjoyed how vinyasa kept you moving. The transitions from pose to pose were fluid with only a few static holds before you moved again. I felt like I got a good workout but I also felt more calm and peaceful by the end of class.

I stuck with yoga, and the girl. Years later we got married, had three beautiful children and together we opened MOSAIC, our own yoga studio. It has been the home for our practice and many others ever since.

For me it all started with a girl. Then it became a new exercise that I loved. Today it is something much, much more.

Since opening MOSAIC a month after completing my 200-hour yoga training in March of 2010, I have taught thousands of classes and tens of thousands of students from a wide variety of backgrounds including professional athletes, special operations military forces and corporate teams. I have taught classes at public studios, at yoga festivals and numerous private functions.

For close to a decade now I have studied yoga's history, philosophy and art. I joke that I got my masters from Amazon because much of what I've learned has been self-taught. While I have had opportunities to train directly with some inspiring teachers, I have spent more hours studying the pages of their books.

The discipline of yoga is a way of life for me. Yoga is no longer an activity that takes place solely during the one hour on my mat. Yoga has slowly transformed my entire being. Bringing my mind, body and spirit into greater alignment with one and other, and with my life as a whole.

I see yoga as the first holistic health coaching program that was ever created, and unlike many others, it not only teaches how to heal the body, but also the mind. Even more than that, it teaches how to connect with your soul. I use the discipline of my practice to inform the discipline of my life. Naturally, the things we become passionate about we want to share with others. I hope that this book can do two things. One, increase your understanding of yoga's rich history, philosophy and science. Two, help you deepen your practice and maybe even ignite the same spark in you, that was ignited in me. The world is full of students, some of whom will rise to be leaders. We call them teachers.

THE EVOLUTION OF A PRACTICE

"Science is progressing. Art is progressing. Yoga as an art and a science, it has to progress. Otherwise there is stagnation again. And someone has to come to life, to revolutionize again." – BKS Iyenar

The growing population of yoga in the West has slowly produced three "camps." The first is focused almost exclusively on the physical postures of asana. Social media is inundated with photos of students and teachers able to move their bodies through gravity defying positions. The second is focused on the philosophy of the practice. They are interested in yoga's traditional roots and how it seeks to answer the mysteries of life. The third is focused on the science. They are interested in studying the claims yoga makes about the mind and body through strict scientific methodologies.

Each of these camps brings an important element, and each one can serve to strengthen the practice of yoga.

Yoga, as Iyengar stated, is both a science and an art – and as such it must evolve. A new generation of practitioners moves in greater force to their mats. They bring with them a desire to be both strong in their bodies and inspired in their lives. Many of them will never study with a teacher who came from the East and they will never venture to India. But that does not deter them. They are excited to gain greater mastery and control over their bodies through the regular practice of asana. They are eager to learn the practices of meditation and mindfulness because they know the benefits they add to living a happy, purpose driven life. They trust the science, but even more than that, they trust their own experiences. They are ready to evolve the science and art of this incredible practice to a living discipline both on and off the mat.

Below is an ethos that I created for our yoga studio. I believe in many ways it captures the beliefs of those who will carry this practice into a new and exciting evolution.

Yogis are. . .

strong, focused, loving, disciplined and **FREE.**

Embrace both flesh and spirit, reason and faith, technology and indigenous wisdom, east and west.

Use their resources to **alleviate the pain** and suffering of others.

Do not practice in front of a mirror because their practice is the mirror. They are **fearless in uncovering their truth** regardless of what they find.

Put **ethics and values** before vanity and glory. They work harder, train harder, and give more on and off their mat.

Use the asana practice not only to **build strength and flexibility** in their body but also in their mind.

Strive to recognize the divine light in all beings and treat each individual with **respect and love**.

Have been tired, injured, broken, and lost but they **always find their way** back to their mat.

Practice with a **peaceful heart and a warrior spirit**.

ONE Focus

ONE Family

ONE Future

ALL IN to Awaken & Uplift

THE HISTORY

THE HISTORY

The Creation Story

In the beginning, there was the Self. One day, before there were any days, the Self had a thought: It thought "I." And as soon as it thought "I" it became afraid. Once you have the thought of existence you are also confronted with the concept of nonexistence. But then the Self reasoned, "Since I am the only one that exists, what is there to be afraid of?" Reassured by this thought, the Self noticed that it was lonely.

So the Self grew until it divided into two, man and woman. As soon as the man and the woman separated, they immediately clung together, as male and female do, and out of this first union came the human race.

After a little while, the female Self thought, "This doesn't seem right. He is like my brother, and I am his sister we are from the same, and so we are the same. He should not attempt to possess me." So, the female Self disengaged and ran away. The male Self ran after her. She hid from him by turning herself into a cow, but he found her, became a bull, and from this union, cattle were created. She thought, "Well, this isn't working!" and ran away again. This time she turned herself into a mare. He found her again, became a stallion and from this union horses were created. She ran again and again, changing from one thing to the next but he still found her until finally the Self looked around and thought, "All this came from me, and I am in all of this."[1]

There are many different creation myths from many different religious and spiritual belief systems. It's important to remember that the creation story is not meant to be taken literally. It is a myth created to give explanation to a subject that is otherwise unexplainable. In this example the myth serves to answer the question, how can God be all knowing, all seeing and a part of everything?

The Gods and Goddesses we sometimes hear referenced in a yoga class often come from the Hindu Mythology epics such as the Mahabharata and Ramayana. Like many myths, they serve to help explain philosophical or moral questions through stories or through what they represent. For example, the Hindu triumvirate consists of three

---

[1] Modified from *From the Gita to the Grail*, by Bernie Clark, along with various other translations [add publisher and date]

gods: Vishnu, Shiva and Brahma. Brahma is the creator of the world, Vishnu is the preserver of the world, and Shiva is the Destroyer - in order for it to be recreated. Together they are **G**enerator, **O**rganizer and **D**estroyer or G.O.D.

The representations of these beings and the moral lessons their stories tell, lend themselves to themes for yoga classes, and so they are found regularly integrated into studio practice.

Hinduism vs. Yoga

Hinduism is the primary belief system of India. Hinduism has many different parts which each emphasize a particular area of study. Yoga is part of Hinduism and is one of the six systems of Hindu philosophy known as darśanas.

Parts of the Hindu Belief System Including Yoga

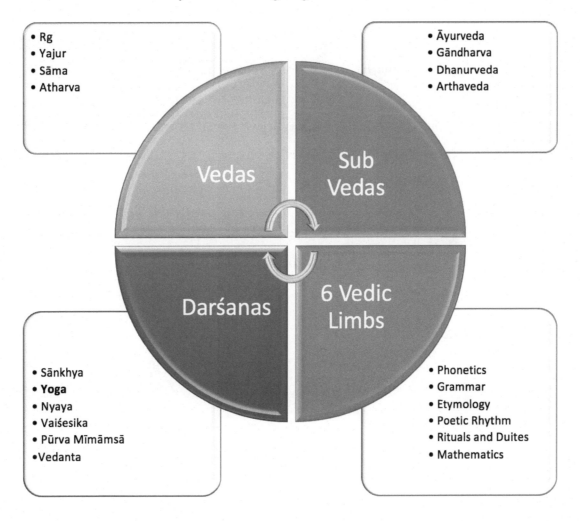

* Rg
* Yajur
* Sāma
* Atharva

* Āyurveda
* Gāndharva
* Dhanurveda
* Arthaveda

Vedas

Sub Vedas

Darśanas

6 Vedic Limbs

* Sānkhya
* **Yoga**
* Nyaya
* Vaiśesika
* Pūrva Mīmāmsā
* Vedanta

* Phonetics
* Grammar
* Etymology
* Poetic Rhythm
* Rituals and Duites
* Mathematics

The six darśanas:

Sānkhya: The distinction between consciousness and nature.

Yoga: The control of the mind that enables one to understand the distinction between consciousness and nature.

Nyāya: Methods of investigating the truth and the discussion of proof.

Vaiśesika: The discussion of various substances found in the universe including atomic theory.

Pūrva Maīmāmsā: The discussion of virtuous conduct and interpretation of Vedic rituals.

Vedānta: The discussion of the nature of God.[2]

Whenever I'm asked the question, "is yoga a religion?" I answer "no."

Yoga is the part of the larger belief system of Hinduism which places emphasis on understanding the mind in a way that allows you to discern between consciousness and nature.

The practice of yoga in the West, is very different from its traditional roots in the East. Through cultural appropriation, yoga has evolved into a practice that relates more to exercise then it does to religion. Parts of yoga have been pulled out, emphasized and positioned as the whole. In particular the practice of asana has become synonymous with the practice of yoga. You will learn in later chapters this is not a fair or accurate synonym.

I believe that yoga is still evolving. While you cannot deny the benefits a regular physical asana practice has for your body, more and more people are starting to embrace the practice as a discipline for spiritual development.

A Great Civilization is Born

Yoga's rich history begins in India close to 6,000 years ago. There, a civilization was born and flourished along the banks of the two main rivers around which it lays, the Indus and Sarasvati.

The Sarasvati River ran through a region located in Pakistan's Sindh province. There, the city of Mohenjo-Daro was built, covering an area nearly 620 acres and serving

---

[2] Ravikanth, *Yoga Sutras of Patanjali*, 2012

as the home to almost 40,000 people. At its center was the citadel located above the lower residential homes. The citadel had a great bath that may have been used for ceremonies or morning prayers.

The residential buildings were constructed of clay bricks. These multi-story buildings had tile bathroom floors, public restrooms, and advanced sewage systems – for their time. The roads were laid out in a geometrical square grid lined with waste receptacles. It was quite easily the biggest civilization in early antiquity.[3]

The people of this city were skilled merchants mastering woodworking, ceramics, brass, and stonework. They appear to have been very peaceful since minimal weapons have been discovered. It also seems that the construction was done without the use of slave labor but in a cooperative way.

Today, only the Indus River remains. The Sarasvati River dried up around 1900 BC, and archeologists think the civilization moved east towards the now well-known Ganges river. No one knows precisely how or why the Sarasvati dried up. Some believe there must have been some tremendous earthquakes or other geographical shift that redirected or disrupted its flow.

Further south along the coast, another city, Dholavira, also thrived. It had a population of roughly 20,000 and during the monsoon season, the people of Dholavira mastered the flow of the river with damns, channeling it into massive reservoirs that surrounded the city. These massive reservoirs were used throughout the year for drinking, washing, cooking and watering crops. The people of Dholavira eventually took to the ocean navigating over 30,000 miles of coastline as they traded goods with neighboring villages and towns.

Other than the fact that these cities were incredible feats of architecture, engineering, construction, and trade, they are also believed to be the birthplace of the Vedas. The Vedas are the four texts that make up the canon of Hinduism. The Rig Veda makes numerous references to the Sarasvati River and is the first place the word yoga is written, as "yuj." There have also been clay seals discovered within the cities which

---

[3] Feuerstein G. P., 2009

appear to depict people seated in the lotus position with legs crossed and arms extended out towards the knees.

There is still much to be learned about these civilizations. The hundreds of images that appear to be a written language have yet to be deciphered, and because so many of the spiritual teachings were passed on in hymnodies (word of mouth), rather than in writing, we don't know much about the details of their lives. While there are many theories, the cause of the decline and ultimate demise of these great cultures after thriving for 500 years is unknown.

The Four Periods of Yoga

1. Archaic Yoga: It is during this time that the four ancient hymnodies, the Vedas (meaning wisdom), and ritual texts of the Aranyakas (forest dwellers) are found. These texts were the "revealed sacred knowledge" from holy people and consisted of thousands of hymns and chants designed to bring good fortune to those who invoked them[4]. They were very ritualistic, and the rituals were not to be performed by just anyone. They were carried out by four priests. Each word and every inflection of tone was believed to be significant, so three would perform the ceremony, while the fourth would observe to make sure each word was spoken correctly and with the right inflection.[5]

2. Pre-classical Yoga: Pre-classical yoga is marked by the Upanishads. The word upanishad means "to come sit near." Students would gather around their teacher to gain their wisdom. The Upanishads took a more philosophical view of life and living. They introduced the concept of reincarnation and an understanding of the energy (chakra) systems in the body. The Upanishads had four central concepts.

1. The ultimate reality of the universe is identical with our innermost nature.
2. Only the realization of this can liberate one from suffering and the necessity of birth, life, and death.
3. One's thoughts and actions determine one's destiny.

---

[4] Feuerstein G. P., 2009

[5] Rosen, 2006

4. Unless one is liberated and achieves formless existence as a result of "true" wisdom, one is reborn.

The most famous of the Upanishads is the Bhagavad-Gītā. It is in this epic Hindu text that the great Lord Krishna reveals the secrets of the universe to Arjuna as he is riding into battle. The Bhagavad-Gītā is also the text which outlines the practices of karma yoga, the discipline of selfless action as the path towards spiritual liberation.

3. Classical Yoga: Classical Yoga is defined by the Yoga Sutras of Patanjali. He wrote his Yoga Sutras around 200 AD. The exact time is difficult to pinpoint as very little is known about Patanjali himself. The word sutra means thread. The sutras consist of 195 aphorisms of yoga wisdom that can easily be committed to memory. Each aphorism is like an individual pearl of wisdom. The pearls can then be threaded together to form a complete philosophical outlook. These aphorisms are divided into four books known as Padas. The Sutras are probably best known in the Western yoga world for the eight limbs outlined as a roadmap for anyone interested in the pursuit of truth. Each limb is designed to help free the practitioner from his or her ignorance (avidya), by revealing a practitioner's true nature (purusa). Among the limbs, you find ethical guidelines for living; breathing techniques; practices for exploring and taming the tumultuous currents of the mind; and of course, the physical practice of yoga postures (asana). Classical yoga is known as yoga Darsana or the philosophical viewpoint. In this era, there are four main paths to God:

1. Karma yoga. The path for the active person, as it is the path of work and duty.
2. Bhakti yoga. The path for the emotional person, as it is the path of devotion and love to a personal God.
3. Jnana yoga. The path of the intellectual person, as it is the path of "right" knowledge.
4. Raja Yoga. The path of the reflective person, as it is the path of controlling the mind and mastering the senses.[6]

---

[6](Iyengar B. , 2005)

It's helpful to think of these four paths as individual colors of a rainbow. Each color mixes and fades into the other creating the complete spectrum of color within light.

4. Post-Classical period: Post-Classical is everything that follows the Yoga Sutras, from about 200 AD onwards. It is at this time that Hatha yoga is born. Hatha means forceful. Hatha yoga places greater emphasis on the purification of the body. Including the physical practice of asanas. Hatha yoga is the foundation for many of the forms of yoga that Westerners practice today, which include: Iyengar, Ashtanga, Vinyasa, Anyasura, Bikram, and Power Yoga.[7]

TKV Krishnamacharya is often given credit for the creation of vinyasa. It has been said that he observed the movements of acrobatics and wrestling and combined them with the poses he was taught by his teacher to develop Suryanamaskara A (Sun Salutations) and the more flowing transitions between postures. In 1933 he opened a yoga shala and trained three teachers who went on to be very influential teachers in the West. They were BKS Iyengar (Iyengar Yoga), Pattabhi Jois (Ashtanga Yoga), and Indra Devi (Vinyasa Yoga).

These four broad categories, from Archaic Yoga to the Post-Classical period, span some 5,000 years. There are many spiritual texts, gurus, and subcategories I did not mention here. My intent with this section is to give you, the reader, a basic understanding of yoga's rich history, and to convey the depth of a practice that is much more than just a one-hour asana class. As a yoga practitioner, you are stepping onto a path that has been walked by many men and women before you. Yoga, whichever path you choose to follow, is not for the weak of heart or faint in spirit. It demands as Iyengar said, "honesty, sustained application and above all love in your heart."

---

[7] (Brooke Boon, 2006)

THE PHILOSOPHY

THE PHILOSOPHY

What is yoga?

The word philosophy comes from the word roots *philo-sophia* meaning *lover of wisdom*. When we study yoga history, listen to teachers, and read books, we gain knowledge. Knowledge is not wisdom. We must seek wisdom through the practical application of knowledge. During that application we must allow for mistakes, and be open to making adjustments. Over time, acting with knowledge, open to learning from experience, we gain wisdom.

Yoga can be said to have many definitions with many different meanings. Like a tree with its roots in India, its branches have grown throughout the world. Today there are many different lineages and styles of yoga. Each style of yoga comes with its own unique exploration of the same core question: who am I?

In Patanjali's Yoga Sutras he defines yoga for us in the second sutra: yogahchittavrttinirodha. Y*oga is the ability to direct the mind exclusively toward an object and sustain that direction without any distractions.*

The word yoga is first written in the Rg Veda as 'yuj,' which means to join, bind, attach or yoke.

We can then say that by stabilizing the fluctuations of the mind, we are able to join the individual parts of the self together to create a complete and true picture of reality. Or as Iyengar once said, "Yoga is the yoking (uniting) of the individual self with the Universal self. It is a practical discipline of the dynamic exposition of thought and life."

What is a yogi?

A yogi is simply one who practices yoga. Another term for a yoga student or spiritual aspirant is sādhaka. A sādhaka more specifically is one who is in the pursuit of merging with the divine source or Brahman.

One definition that I particularly like comes from BKS Iyengar.

"[A yogi] uses all his resources – physical, economic, mental or moral – to alleviate the pain and suffering of others. He shares his strength with the weak until they become strong. He shares his courage with those that are timid until they become brave by his example. He denies the maxim of the 'survival of the fittest', but makes the weak strong enough to survive. He becomes a shelter to one and all." – *Light on Yoga*, BKS Iyengar

By this definition, a yogi is a leader. One who through austerity, their own will, and a surrender to God, is driven to serve others and the world with a peaceful heart and a warrior spirit. The path of the yogi is not for the weak minded or the weak willed. It is for those who know deep down that there is a wellspring of potential that has yet to be discovered and they simply need a discipline to help them discover it.

Human development towards a spiritual life

The human brain has evolved quite a bit from its primitive ancestors. One model of this evolution is the triune brain. As you may have guessed from the name, it has three parts.

The oldest part of our brain is the reptilian brain. It is composed of our brain stem and spinal cord and includes the cerebellum which controls balance, reflexes, and movement. The primary function of the reptilian brain is to feed, flee, fornicate and fight. At this level, there are no emotional disturbances to these acts. An example I often give to students is this. Imagine an alligator swimming around a small section of a swamp. One day a much larger alligator slowly swims past the smaller alligator and then continues on its way. The smaller alligator does not spend the rest of the day worrying about the larger alligator. He does not think to himself, "Is he coming back? Why was he swimming so slow? I bet he wants my area of the swamp. I could take him. Could I? Maybe I should call some of my other alligator buddies in case he does come back."

If the larger alligator were to have shown aggression one would win out over the other and that would be the end of it. They would both go about their days looking for something to eat and when the season was right, find a mate to reproduce.

The second level of the triune brain is the mammalian brain. This is our limbic system. It is responsible for such things as language, emotions and memory. It is at this level of evolution that we develop an understanding of hierarchy, status, and communities. Robert Sapolsky, researcher and author of *Why Zebras Don't Get Ulcers,* explains the stress responses in the animals that he has studied in terms of their limbic system.

Research has shown that a regular meditation practice affects this area of the brain, helping to reduce fear and anxiety and improving memory.

The third brain is the neocortex or human brain. The neocortex is the most recent evolution of the brain and is responsible for executive functions, intellectual reasoning, discernment, conscious thought and self-awareness. It is at this level that we have the ability to reflect upon our own existence and can ponder upon the concept of spirituality.

While having brains that have evolved over two million years of evolution has its benefits, it does not come without a price. With the ability to ignore primal instincts, we become subject to the polarities of pleasure and pain. We experience suffering through a constant need to "improve our status" in a variety of ways and means.

At some point in human history, a desire to alleviate suffering became a priority. Human beings were then driven towards the pursuit of the highest ideal, God (Isvara) to focus their attention. Through this process an ethical and moral code of conduct (yamas and niyamas) was developed, to live in greater harmony with nature, fellow human beings and oneself. The peak of this was the ability to live in line with the ideals of God and independent of race, class or faith.

Duty, Wealth, Pleasure and Liberation

In yoga philosophy, there are four aims in life, these are known as the purusārthas.

Dharma

Dharma is defined as duty and ethical discipline. There are two types of dharma. The first is our own personal dharma. It is the application of our individual gifts, talents and skills in service to others and our community. This dharma is unique to us and sometimes needs to be discovered through introspection and self-reflection. The second type is universal dharma. This is the universal code that governs "right" action. Classical yoga gives us the yamas and niyamas as foundational guidelines from which to act in accordance with dharma. (The yamas and niyamas are explained in detail later).

Artha

Artha is the word to describe the acquisition of wealth. In yoga teacher training many students are surprised to see that the generation of wealth is listed as an aim in life. Wealth in and of itself is not good or bad. It is both the attitude and emotion that we assign to it, and the actions that we use it for, that create problems. Ideally, wealth should be generated in order to allow for independence and higher pursuits. You will see in the next section that a student progresses slowly towards dedicating more and more of their time to their awakening. It becomes obvious then that we must have enough money to support us later in life or we will still be required to be very much "in the world" as we will need to continue to work to make money to support ourselves.

Kama

Kama is experiencing the pleasures of life through a healthy body. Many people are often surprised by this concept as well. You may even have heard that, when it comes to the spiritual life, physical pleasure is seen as creating suffering and should not be a focus at all, let alone an aim in life. It is not pleasure itself that is harmful, it is our unhealthy attachments to that pleasure and the waterfall of effects those attachments have on our overall happiness.

Imagine you work a 9-5 job that you don't love. It's Sunday evening and the last day of your Hawaii vacation. Tomorrow you have to fly back to your normal routine, and to work. You're sitting on the beach watching the sunset. taking in the beauty of the moment. You feel relaxed and at peace. Then you start to think about how you have to leave in the morning. You start to think that in a few more minutes the sun will fall below the horizon and that this is the end of your vacation. The final few moments of experiencing the pleasure of the sunset are lost because they were spent dreading the future. You're grappling to hold onto something that will never last. This is what creates suffering.

The pleasures of a physical life should be kept in check and not made into the primary focus of our existence. If we do focus on them, they become indulgences, and our identity and sense of self gets entangled in them. In extreme cases, we become hedonistic, constantly craving and desiring for more pleasure, while at the same time fearing the lack of it. Instead, spiritual pursuits should be our primary focus. The goal is to achieve liberation from our ego-mind, transcending into a new understanding of self. That process, however, is done in a physical body and there is nothing wrong with allowing physical pleasures to exist as long as they do not control us. We have to learn to be masters of our senses instead of slaves to them.

Moksa

The final aim of one's life is liberation. Liberation is the ability to free oneself from the false understanding of identity as ego, and to embrace the truth of the human soul and the completeness of your own divine nature. In yoga, this is the ultimate aim of one's life. Dharma, Artha, and Kama all help to achieve this aim. Dharma, ethical discipline, is required as a foundation for correct living in hopes of achieving liberation. Artha is the acquisition of wealth that give us the financial support we need later in our life to be able to pursue liberation without financial worry or the need to participate actively in an of the world job. Kama teaches us to distinguish between physical pleasure and spiritual understanding so we can begin to release our attachments to the need to appease our mind and senses. When one achieves the state of Moksha, one is free.

4 Stages of life (āśrama):

According to yoga philosophy, there are four stages to a person's life: brahmacharaya grihastha, vanaprastha and sannyasa. To best outline them I've first provided a brief explanation of each and then elaborated with reflections upon my own personal experiences. My reason for this is to give you a look at how each stage is relevant even today.

As a man, a business owner and a father, I don't fit the stereotypical Western profile of a yogi, but I am one, or at least trying to be one. Yoga has shaped who I am as a parent, a partner and a businessman. Owning and operating two yoga studios on opposite coasts while being present for my kids and wife has its challenges. Through it all I have relied on the teachings of yoga to guide me through the ups and downs of the various stages I find myself at. Here's how.

The first stage (brahmacharaya) is that of a child and a student. In this stage you're learning the world around you and understanding your place in it. There is particular emphasis on the higher virtues of compassion, understanding, respect, justice and integrity.

The second stage (grihastha) is that of the householder. This is the time of finding a partner and raising a family. Additionally, this stage is a time to build wealth through your career path of choice. However, it's important to note that it is never done at the expense of the lessons learned in the first stage.

The third stage (vanaprastha) is the time of retirement. This is traditionally thought to begin when your children are old enough to get married and begin their own families. It is at this stage that you shift your focus towards your spiritual maturation, setting aside material goals for the higher pursuits of self-knowledge.

The final stage (sannyasa) is the stage of renunciation. It is a time to release worldly desires for the full efforts of spiritual awakening.

This is not to say that one should wait until our golden years to begin our yoga practice, but more to highlight that yoga recognizes that life is full of responsibilities and duties; that these duties vary in focus at different times in our lives and, most importantly, that yoga can help you navigate each one of them with more strength (stihram) and ease (sukham).

STAGE 1 Brahmacharya (the student)

My early years of development have past, but those of my children have not. My wife and I have always felt that early childhood development was one of the most important stages of a person's life and so we've looked to yoga and other philosophies like it to help guide us as we raise our kids during these early years. Our girls know that Mommy and Daddy have time to pray and meditate. They started working on their Down Dogs with

Daddy at the same time they started learning to walk. They know we have a strong faith in God and that we believe in an eternal soul that progresses from one life to the next.

My oldest daughter is now seven and is homeschooled. When she was younger she went to a school that fit with our beliefs. In our search we came across the Waldorf school, started by the philosopher Rudolf Steiner. One of Waldorf's key tenets is "Do no harm to others, do no harm to yourself and do no harm to the environment." Children are taught to live in harmony with nature and each other before ever asked to read and write. Similarly, the yamas of Patanajali's *Yoga Sutras* state that one should do no harm, be honest, not steal or take what isn't ours, that one should restrain from sexual misconduct, and should not long for more than we need. The Waldorf system allows kids to develop together and teaches about the intimate and important relationship we have with the earth, each other and ourselves. We believe that learning these principles now builds the foundation for great success as our daughter progresses through the remaining three stages of her life.

STAGE 2 Grihastha (the householder)

I find myself in this stage. I have been married for 10 years now to the most amazing woman. I have three beautiful children and am the co-founder of MOSAIC. Along with my wife and a mutual friend, I started MOSAIC in a 400 square foot upstairs apartment in San Diego, California. At the same time, my wife and I began plans for our family. Within a year we had been fortunate enough to expand and took on an additional 700 square foot space in the same building. It wasn't long after that my first daughter, Leela, was born. A couple years later, with a growing yoga community, we had an opportunity to expand our business again by taking on a new location of roughly 2,100 square feet. During that process my second daughter, Carin, was born. A few years later we moved to the other side of the country to Virginia and opened the doors to our second studio in Charlottesville. While there we had our third child, a boy named Gabriel. Two years later we moved back to San Diego and as I write this we are preparing to be foster parents for infants.

The mission of MOSAIC has taken on different words from time to time but it has always been the goal to provide a space where people could awaken and uplift their soul.

We also opened it with the hope that owning our own business would allow us flexibility in our schedules to have one or both of us home with our kids all the time. We are very blessed that this has proven to be true and we have been able to spend so much time with our kids through the earliest years of their lives. The conclusion of this stage will see my kids grown and ready to begin their own families. My hope is that at the same time we will have built a business that they can step into running with the fresh spirit of their youth.

STAGE 3 Vanaprastha (retirement)

With only 36 years of life under my belt I've yet to reach this third stage. Because of this I lack a certain wisdom of what it will bring. What I hope and plan is that this stage of life will be a time to mindfully transition from a focus of worldly acquisitions to spiritual ones. If I'm lucky my children will have taken enough interest in MOSAIC and the services we have provided to want to lead the business in a more active role. For me, Vanaprastha will be a time to become an advisor to my kids while I focus on the "inner limbs" in Patanjali's Yoga Sutras. These limbs: Pratayahara, Dharana, Dhyana, and Samadhi are a progression from the withdrawal of the senses from the outside world, to a state of concentration, through a state of meditation, and finally into a state of enlightenment.

STAGE 4 Sannyasa (renunciation)

The yogic view of life is a bit different from that of the typical American. Instead of viewing the years after retirement as a slow decline of one's health and influence in the world, the yogi sees the third and fourth stages as the most important. This is the time for ascension of the mind back to the soul. In the sannyasa stage all energy is given to one's spiritual work. In this stage my role will be to serve as an example to my children and grandchildren on the natural evolution of a life centered on healthy, wise, spiritual principles. In this way, I hope they may find inspiration and confidence in their abilities to do the same.

There is no doubt that the past 10 years have been busy. My discipline has waxed and waned at times but it has always been there in some fashion. I often times reflect back on the four stages of the yogi's life when I feel I am behind in my efforts or questioning a business or parenting decision. I find them to be a comfort in letting me know there's still plenty of time for my spiritual maturation. They make me want to rise to the challenge to do the work necessary to be a role model for my children, grandchildren and anyone who wants a life in the world that is spiritually focused. I am continuously humbled by the work that lies ahead of me while encouraged by the many blessings the yoga discipline has provided.

Who Am I? Nature, Soul, and God

At the most basic level, there are three fundamental components. They are Prakrti, Purusa and Isvara.

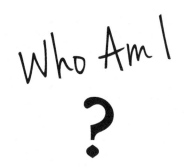

Prakrti is the matter which makes up the physical universe, from the smallest particle to the largest star. Prakrti is embodied, to varying degrees, by three separate elements. These elements give all form certain qualities. These three elements are collectively referred to as the Gunas. The three Gunas are rajas (action), tamas (inertia), and sattva (illumination).

Similar to Chinese medicine's yin and yang, rajas and tamas represent the two polar spectrums of energy. The balance of these energies is sattva.

Since the mind is also part of Prakrti, it too is subject to the influences of rajas, tamas and sattva. The ideal state of mind is that of sattva.

A great analogy that I've found comes from B. Ravikanth's book, *Yoga Sutras of Patanjali*. In it he explains the three Gunas in this way:

Imagine you wanted to write something on a whiteboard with a marker. The marker is like sattva. Without it nothing can be written or understood. The hand is like rajas. If the hand does not move then nothing can be written. The whiteboard is like tamas. A stable surface is needed to write on. If any of these are out of balance – the hand moves too quickly, the marker is out of ink or the board is wobbly – then one cannot write effectively.

The second fundamental element is Purusa. Purusa is the name for each individual soul. It is sometimes refered to as Atman. Every living being is a Purusa. There are innumerable numbers of Purusas and all but one are on a journey of self-discovery.

The one Purusa that is not on this journey is Isvara. Isvara is the word for Lord or God in Sanskrit. God has three very important qualities that differentiate it from all other Purusas. God is omniscient, omnipotent, and omnipresent. God does not need nature to know anything; God knows everything by God's very nature.[8] God makes use of matter to create the environment for individual souls to access the knowledge and wisdom of their true nature.

The Divine Movement Toward Life

In their primordial state, the three Gunas are perfectly balanced with none more dominant than another. This completely balanced state is like standing in the dark, of a pitch black room full of furniture. You can see no differentiation of objects, only the darkness. If I were to ask you to point to a single piece of furniture in the room and describe its attributes it would be impossible. This is the primordial state of the Gunas.

In order for consciousness to attain knowledge, it needs differentiation. If there was not hot, you could not know cold. If there was not up, you could not know down. If there was no bad, you could not know good. In this way, if there is no form you cannot know soul.

So, God turned on the lights, and influenced the ratio of rajas, tamas and sattva, starting off a chain of events that set the evolution of prakrti into motion. Eventually leading to human beings.

The first movement or evolute is called Mahat. It is the creation of buddhi, the intellect.

The second evolute is the formation of Ahankāra, the ego. Ahankāra is then sub-divided into two parts: sattva-dominated and tamas-dominated.

From the sattva-dominated ego comes three things.

---

[8] (Ravikanth, 2012)

1. The five subtle instruments of knowledge: hearing, touching, seeing, tasting, and smelling.
2. The five subtle instruments of action: speech, grasping, locomotion, excretion, and gratification.
3. The mind. The mind is the coordinator of these ten senses as well as being the source of desire and impulse.

From tamas-dominated ego comes two things.
1. The foundation for the five subtle elements of sound, touch, sight, taste, and smell
2. The five elements of nature: space, air, fire, water, and earth

Everything with a physical form comes from the five elements of nature: the mineral kingdom, the plant kingdom, and the animal kingdom, eventually evolving to human beings.

With this new understanding, let us come back to the big question: who am I? Simply put, you are Purusa, but it's more complex than that.

Let's call Purusa pure consciousness. This consciousness is not physical in form and is separate from, yet connected to, the mind.

The mind is often referred to as chitta. From my research, chitta appears to be interpreted as a combination of the mind, the intellect and the ego all wrapped into one. Chitta combined with the five subtle elements of perception and the five subtle elements of action makes up the subtle body.

When our physical body dies, the subtle body, connected to our higher consciousness, moves into a new body, taking with it the impressions from the previous life. Some of those impressions may be active but most are inactive which is why we cannot remember our previous life memories. It has been said, however, that mastered yogis can call upon their previous life memories and experiences.

When in physical form, the subtle body is connected to the gross body. The gross body is composed of the five external organs of perception and action.
They are as follows:

External Sense Organs: ears, skin, eyes, tongue, and nose

External Motor Organs: tongue, hands, legs, genitals, and excretory organs

The physical body is of course more intricate than this, and composed of much more, but this list highlights the connections between the subtle and physical sense organs as viewed from yoga philosophy.

The soul (Purusa) is then born into a physical body which exists in a physical space (Prakrti). The physical world is highly differentiated. The physical world is defined by a pair of extreme opposites and any number of variations between those two extremes.

The soul uses the body and senses as a mechanism to realize its true nature so that it can eventually return back to its state of Purusa with the wisdom of its divine nature intact. This takes many lifetimes. The exact number of lifetimes is unknown because the work that we do in any given lifetime can influence how quickly we progress towards an enlightened awareness.

In summary, Purusa, the universal self, gives way to Prakrti, physical form. The mix of these energies creates the five elements of earth, water, air, fire and space, and their five subtle counterparts of smell, taste, form, touch and sound. Anything with a physical form contains varying degrees of the three Gunas. In this way consciousness creates matter; matter does not create consciousness.

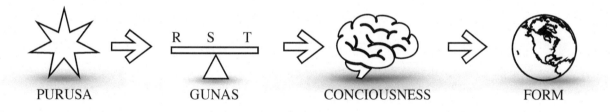

PURUSA   GUNAS   CONCIOUSNESS   FORM

The Sheaths of Self

There are five layers or sheaths of the human being, they are known as the Kosas. The five Kosas are as follows: Physical sheath – Anamaya kosa, Energetic sheath – Pranamaya Kosa, Mental sheath – Manamaya Kosa, Intellectual sheath – Vjnayama Kosa, and Divine sheath – Anandamaya Kosa.

The sheaths are sometimes compared to a Russian Doll or the layers of an onion. You can also think of them like the varying spectrums of light through a prism.

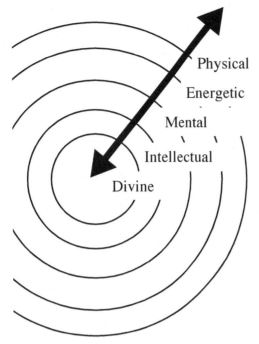

Physical
Energetic
Mental
Intellectual
Divine

When you shine a beam of light, there is no telling where the red light wave is vs. the blue or green, etc. It is a single white beam of light. But when you pass it through a prism, the light is fractured and split into its different waves of color. In goes white light, out comes a rainbow. Think of the prism like your yoga practice. You pass your light through your practice so you can see and work with each of the varying layers of yourself more clearly, and with more precision.

Anamaya Kosa — Physical: Through the practice of postures you stretch certain muscles and strengthen others. Your nervous system is toned through an appropriately sequenced yoga class by adding stress (sympathetic activation) and relaxation (parasympathetic activation). Your bones and joints are strengthened by applying proper load and by moving them through full ranges of motion. When practiced correctly, the asana is balanced between stihra and sukha. These somewhat opposing forces keep the asana balanced between effort and comfort. When mindfully moving in asana you may feel the difference between one side and the other, noticing the asymmetry that exists in your body, and thus, be able to work with the body to bring it back to symmetry. You can become more aware of your body's habit patterns and consciously choose if the pattern you are caught in is the appropriate movement for you given the time and conditions. All of these things and more can be learned when we apply the principles of yoga to our asana practice, giving us greater insight into our physical sheath as we continue to refine and develop its health and balance.

The physical sheath must also be kept healthy for Kama, a healthy body is necessary for enjoying the physical pleasures of life. More detail on Kama can be found in the earlier section entitled: Duty, Wealth, Pleasure, and Liberation.

Pranamaya Kosa – Energy: When you practice the breathing techniques of pranayama, you are working more closely with Pranamaya Kosa, the energy sheath. Prana is life force energy. Pranayama is the manipulation of breath to actively manipulate the movement of energy through the body. The breath is the subtlest part of the physical body and the coarsest part of the subtle body.[9] It is therefore the bridge between the two. When combined with asana you not only move the energy but you clear the nadis, the channels that energy moves through. The folding, twisting, and extending of the body from pose to pose helps to open the nadis and allow for pranic energy to move with greater ease. You can also consciously work to bring energy to a particular chakra center by focusing on drawing the energy in towards Sushumna, the center energy nadi that runs in line with the spine.

I always teach that we have to learn to move the breath around the body and then move the body around the breath. What do I mean by this? When we are practicing pranayama, we are not just breathing in and out air. We are moving energy. In this way, energy is not restricted to the lungs and upper thoracic cavity. Prana moves everywhere and is said to flow with more intensity in the areas that our minds are focused on. When breathing in your yoga practice, breathe with your entire body. Focus the mind on the areas that the asana calls it to. Listen and adjust. Learn to create the adjustment around the movement of the breath.

Manamaya Kosa – Mental: When you do a yoga pose it does not just happen in your body. It is the mind that tells the body where to go in the first place. The mind says, "Put your foot between your hands, spin your back heel down and lift up into Warrior II." Then, your mind, if left unexamined, may decide that Warrior II is uncomfortable so you don't like it, or that it doesn't feel as strong as it did yesterday, so you are upset that you feel weak. The mind wants to feel pleasurable, or at the very least satiated. You can use your asana practice to work with both the mind and the intellectual sheaths here.

If you've been practicing yoga for a while, when your mind moves the body into a position that it is familiar with, it tends to go on autopilot, based off of a motor program it has created through the repetition of that movement over a period of time. This is referred to as "chunking." It was discovered when researchers at MIT started to test the basal ganglia in rats asked to carry out a simple and repetitive task. What they noticed was the more the rat carried out the task the less brain activity could be observed. What

---

[9] (Powers, 2008)

seemed to take over was the basal ganglia, a lump of tissue found in the brains of humans, mammals and reptiles .[10]

Chunking is a mechanism for energy efficiency and it explains why you brush your teeth the same way every night without having to think about the action. The same holds to a regular asana practice. The mind will repeat the pattern it has learned and then it may take a step further and pass judgment on the pose, how it feels, compare it to your expectations for yourself and determine if the experience is pleasurable or not. If the mind is pleased, it is more likely to want to repeat. If not, then the opposite holds true.

Vjnamaya Kosa – Intellect: The intellectual sheath is crucial to your yoga practice. This layer of self can look at the pose and the habit patterns of the body with a discerning eye. The intellectual sheath can examine a pose free of emotional attachments or entanglements with one's ego. This is mindfulness, and it brings us into the present moment and the pose at hand. As Iyengar once said, "I practice the pose of today, not yesterday, and not tomorrow." The intellectual sheath is more objective, whereas the mental sheath is more subjective. I teach that the first breath in a pose is the habit. It is the position that we take because we have been there before. The body knows the motions. The second breath is where we engage the intellectual sheath. We see the pose for what it is, and we have the insight of what might need to be adjusted. The third breath is action. It is the opportunity to choose consciously what to change and how to move forward.

Anandamaya Kosa – Divine: The divine sheath is the final layer. It is the return to the soul. It is the layer where there is no time and no comparisons. Our ego lives on comparisons; comparison to others, to different situations and even to ourselves. It is in the sheath of the soul that we are free. Imagine a space in your mind where your thoughts are not making any comparisons. Even the contrast between thought and non-thought is a comparison. The final sheath is a return home to the true nature of the self. It is the ray of light that carries on lifetime after lifetime until we know so clearly that it is us, that we were never anything else.

---

[10] (Duhigg, 2012)

The practice of yoga was designed to break us free of the ego mind construct by purifying all layers while simultaneously penetrating from the outer layer of the physical self to the inner layer of the divine self.

The Natural State of Suffering

All human beings, with the exception of maybe a few who were born enlightened, experience suffering. The Sanskrit word for suffering is dhukha, and defined as the quality of mind that leaves us feeling squeezed. It does not necessarily relate to physical pain, it is a tension or pain in the mind.[11] Dhukha plays out in many ways in our lives but is said to arise most when we try to rush our development, cannot adjust to new situations, or when we try to change old habits.

When we are born into a body, we lose our awareness of our Purusa (true) nature. The physical brain and mind build a construct of reality in order to be able to place ourselves within that reality. We slowly develop an ego that is fed by both nature and nurture. At about 18 months of age sensations are not just sensations but something that is happening to "me". Eg: I'm hot or I'm hungry. This I, me, ego, separates us even further from our true nature and from each other.

The Sanskrit term for this ignorance of our true nature is avidya. Avidya is fed by four other aspects of our personalities. They are: the ego itself, unreasonable wants and desires, rejections of things based on past experiences, and fear. Avidya, supports and perpetuates dhukha.

Ego (Asmitā): The ego is the identity construct that is built by the mind in order to be able to place itself within its environment. We see everything as separate from us. The ego is in a constant comparison, always looking and judging ourselves against others. The ego is also constantly fighting for its preservation and does not like to be wrong. We've all been in the situation where we get into an argument, and somewhere between the back and forth you realize that the person you're arguing with is actually right and you're wrong. But for some reason you don't just admit this. Instead you continue to argue your point even when you are now consciously aware that you are

---

[11] (Desikachar, The Heart of Yoga: Developing A Personal Practice, 1999)

wrong! Why do we do it? Because the ego hates to be wrong. Why is that? Because if we are wrong then we might compare ourselves unfavorably to the person who is right, and emotionally we want to protect ourselves from that.

Wants (Rāga): The mind is influenced heavily by our senses. What we see, hear, taste, touch, and smell registers as either a good sensation, a bad sensation, or a neutral sensation. If the sensation is good we want to repeat it. If it's really good we want to repeat it even more. One of my teachers, Jim Cahill, refers to the mind as your unethical personal assistant. It asks you, "Are you going to do this again tomorrow?" If the answer is yes, then it will make it easier for you. If you continue to answer yes, you eventually won't even have to think about it . . . and it will be really hard to stop. This is how habits are formed. It is unethical because it doesn't stop to think whether the action is good or bad – that's the job of the intellect. It's only interested in immediate gratification. When we cannot repeat a "good" sensation we become frustrated, disappointed, angry, even depressed. We might even not be able to enjoy a positive sensation because we are thinking about it being over and maybe not getting it again. It sounds crazy when it's written down like this but it's true. Have you ever had a Monday-Friday, 9-5 job? If so, can you remember Sunday? You could spend half of a great Sunday thinking about how it was going to be Monday tomorrow and you had to go back to work. Sunday night blues robs you of almost a quarter of your weekend.

Rejections (Dvesa): When we experience negative sensations, we seek to avoid them. From the position of evolution this was an important mechanism for survival. If you went exploring the cave of a saber tooth tiger once, your brain would remember its location so that you didn't go back again. But, what about in non-life threatening situations?

Have you ever been so upset after a break-up that you said, "I'm never dating again! I'd rather be alone!" We shouldn't throw the baby out with the bath water because if we do we may miss out on a really great life experience, and an important opportunity to grow.

Fear (Abhiniveśa): Of all the limbs of Avidya, fear is the biggest contributor to our ignorance. There are plenty of non-mortal fears that we all experience. Judgements, uncertainty, change, financial stability, being alone, not achieving our potential. Can you relate to any of those? Of course you can. We all can. Every teacher training, I have the class write down some of their non-mortal fears and then share them, and every time they are the same. When we start to peel back some of the layers, we are not so different from one another.

From a spiritual view however, it is the fear of death that is the greatest contributor to our ignorance. To the mastered yogi, death is like taking off an old coat. The soul lives on just as vibrant as it has always been. Death is simply a transition from one place to another. When we know this not just as a concept, but as an experience of our being, we are free.

Karma & Reincarnation

Karma means action. When a rock is dropped into a still lake, ripples created by the rock radiate out towards the shore. When they hit the shore, they reverse back towards the rock. Karma operates in much the same way. Actions which create karma ripple out into the world. Eventually they will come back, in some shape or form, in order for our soul to learn a lesson.

Let's say for example you rob from people in this lifetime. In a future lifetime you may experience being robbed. Both experiences have something different to teach the soul, so both are important.

When we think, feel, or act in a way that is aligned with the afflictions to consciousness just explained, we can generate karma.

Each life we also bring with us any karma that we left unresolved from previous lifetimes. One of the goals of yoga is to clear our karmic inheritance from past lives and to stop generating new karma in this one.

In any given moment your Karma exists in four different states. Those states are: fully active, blocked, restrained or dormant.

The current events of our lives, along with our current level of awareness, shift our karma into these different states.

In order to stop producing karma we have to teach ourselves to align our thoughts, feelings and actions to our Soul and not to our ignorance. This is a long and slow process which is why it takes lifetimes to achieve.

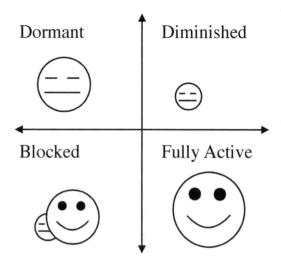

How does one clear their karma? I will share what my teachers have shared with me. There are two parts. The first is choice. We have to make better choices as to where we place our focus. This comes through the process of discernment. The second is will. We must use our will to live our choices through action. Both are necessary, and both can be weak. We can make poor choices but have a strong will or we could make great choices but have a weak will. Through the practice of yoga we must improve our choices and strengthen our will.

Reincarnation is the natural process of being born into new lifetimes over and over again. Its function is to allow the soul time to perfect all that it needs, in order to come to its full awareness and truth. There is simply too much for the soul to learn in one lifetime, so it must continue to come back until it is no longer necessary.

Yoga and Your Mind

The mind is what occupies it. By this definition, if the mind were to be free of preoccupations, would it cease to exist? The concept of mind is a tricky one. Our conscious thoughts are simple enough to recognize, but what about our subconscious mind? We have beliefs, habits, and paradigms built over time that shape and color the way we experience the present moment. Do we actually have free will? Some researchers suggest that we do not. Instead they argue that our perceived conscious choices were already made by our subconscious mind without us knowing, and we are simply carrying out the subconscious decision. While the in-depth study of the mind is fascinating, it is also quite complex and not the focus of this book, so in this section we will look at the mind from the perspective of classical yoga.

We are constantly inundated with thoughts all day, with some sources suggesting we have as many as 60,000. We can categorize these thoughts into five different activities of the mind.

Comprehension

Comprehension is achieved in three ways: direct perception, inference and testimony.[12] Direct perception is when the mind has a direct experience with the object of its attention and it is able to gather information about that object. For example, if I were to set an orange down in front of you, you would be able to see its color, size, and texture. If you were to pick it up you would gain knowledge about its weight. If you were to peel it and eat it, you would learn about its smell and taste. Each of these activities would increase your comprehension of the orange. Inference is if you were to taste the orange juice directly from the orange and at a later date be served it in a glass. After drinking the juice from the glass, you could infer it came from an orange. Testimony occurs when listening to a trusted source or expert on the object of our attention. If I were talking to an orange farmer I trusted and they were to explain facts about oranges to me, I would accept their explanation.

Misapprehension

Misapprehension is when we think we have comprehension but new information leads us to understand that we were in some way wrong, or didn't have the full picture. For example, if you were to see a smaller orange that had not fully ripened, you would see that it is small and yellow. You might think it were a lemon. Upon further exploration, you could discern that it is in fact an orange and so you would have misapprehended the object originally.

Imagination

This is when the mind imagines things that do not exist (vastuśūnya). This happens when, for example, you visualize an orange and then imagine it sprouting legs and arms

---

[12] (Ravikanth, 2012)

and walking around. Your imagination has created a mental image of something that does not exist in reality.

Deep Sleep

I have seen this activity of the mind explained in two different ways so I will include each. The first is the state in which the mind is void of any conscious thoughts because it is engaged in a state of dreamless sleep. While there is no conscious awareness of mind there is still some activity. The second explanation for deep sleep defines it not as sleep, but as the moment that we become aware that we were in an unconscious sleep state but having that awareness means that we are no longer in that state.

Memory

This is the non-loss of impressions of direct experiences. Our interactions with the world creates impressions on the mind. Depending on the experience, these impressions may exist in our short-term memory or our long-term memory. Either way this is the activity of the mind that calls up the mental images of the past event. This is not a reliable source of truth because a memory can never be proven or disproven as true. This is because it exists only in your own mind and your life experiences color the events of reality with our own biases. Two people can have a same experience with a very different memory of it.

These five activities of the mind do not exist independently. Think of it instead as an interconnected web with any one taking more dominance over another at any given moment.

The mind, influenced by the limbs of ignorance, fluctuates between different states. Yoga identifies five main states. It is possible to have an almost infinite number of permutations of these five states. These five states are: Mudha, Ksipta, Viksipta, Ekagra, and Niruddha.

Mudha (stupefied): The ability to observe, act and react is not present. This could be seen as the opposite extreme of Ksipta. Mudha can be affected by diet and lifestyle choices. The Mudha mind is perceived as heavy or depressed. The animal that is often associated with this state of mind is the water buffalo.

Ksipta (scattered, restless): Thoughts, feelings, emotions, and perceptions come and go like waves in a rapid. A Ksipta mind finds it hard to sustain focus. The animal association with this state of mind is a drunken monkey.

Viksipta (distracted): Activity is taking place but it lacks specific purpose and direction. We might be swinging between knowing what one wants to uncertainty. This state of mind is like a slow swinging pendulum. In yoga, this is said to be the most common state of mind.

Ekagra (focused, one-pointed): The mind is now clear and with direction. The mind now has the ability to stay focused in one direction and move forward with attentiveness. When Ekagra is fully developed, it peaks at the fifth and final level, Niruddha.

Niruddha (restrained): The mind is completely linked with the object of its attention. Eventually the mind and object merge into one. This is also a state of Dahrana (more on Dharana later) which when developed leads us to Samadhi.

The five states of the mind should be and are different from the five activities of the mind. For example, one can have comprehension of an object through direct perception but be unable to focus on the object for long because the mind is in a state of ksipta.

The practice of yoga is one that systematically brings a practitioner from a distracted state of mind to an attentive one. How this is achieved is explained in the following section.

The Path to Joy

All of the moments of your life have had an influence on how you view yourself, the world and others. In yoga, this sum of events is called Samskara. Yoga asks us to be more conscious with our actions so that Samskara may have a positive influence on us. Purusa is experienced by means of the mind. If the mind is clear, our powers of observation are clear. If the mind is colored, then our perceptions are colored. Yoga clears the lense of consciousness so that as Iyengar once said, "Our divine light can easily shine out, and the light of god can shine in."

Before we can take any steps towards freedom from suffering, we have to first recognize and admit that it exits. Awareness is the first step towards freedom from Dhukha. This awareness however can unfortunately, at first, lead to more suffering before it leads to more peace. The simple fact is that someone seeking clarity will always be more sensitive to hardships and suffering because their eyes are open to them. A perfect quote to express this comes from Vyasa's commentary on the Yoga Sutras, where he writes, "Dust that lands on the skin is harmless, but if only a tiny particle gets into the eye, it is very painful."

In Patanjali's Yoga Sutras we are given a road map away from suffering and towards freedom. This map is often referred to as the 8-limbed path. Each limb, while able to stand alone, is part of the whole and needs to be cultivated in conjunction with the other limbs to be successful. The eight limbs are yama, niyama, asana, pranayama, pratayahara, dharana, dhyana, and Samadhi. I have detailed each below.

The 8 Limbs of Yoga

1. YAMA

The five virtues that govern our relationships with others and the world.

1. Ahimsa: Loving kindness, embracing flow of nature, compassion, mercy, and gentleness. Non-violence.

2. Satya: Being genuine and authentic to our inner nature. Not lying, downplaying, or exaggerating.

3. Asteya: Not taking what is not yours (money, goods, credit). Not robing people of their expereince and freedom.

4. Brahmacarya: Acting with unconditional love and integrity without selfishness or manipulaiton. Sexual responsibility, not lusting.

5. Aparigraha: Eliminating possessiveness, covetousness and attachment to things. Fostering simplicity and possession of things based only on their functionality.

2. NIYAMA

The five observances relating to one's own physical appearance, actions, words and thoughts that govern our relationship with ourselves.

1. Sauca: Cleanliness, precision, clarity, balance. Internal and external purification.

2. Santosha: Equanimity, peace, tranquility, acceptance of the way things are.

3. Tapas: Burning desire for understanding the higher awareness expressed through self-discipline, purification, will power, austereity and patience.

4. Svadhyaya: Self-inquiry, mindfulness, study of wisdom literature.

5. Ishvara Pranidhana: Faith, trust, open-heartedness, love. "Not my will, but thy will be done." Service and surrender to God. Selfless action.

3. ASANA

The postures for creating strength of body, steadiness of intelligence, and benevolence of spirit. The modern day understanding of asana is different from its traditional roots in classical yoga. In Patanjali's Sutras asana is only mentioned twice and references a single position.

Today asana is understood to be the name given for the multitude of physical postures we commonly practice in a yoga class. This evolution happened over time with a majority of the postural exercise first developing in Hatha Yoga .[13]

4. PRANAYAMA

Pranayama has already been covered in great detail in earlier sections of this book so I will simply summarize here. Prana is the word for life force energy. Pranayama is the title for the many breathing practices designed to help the yogi master life force energy.

5. PRATAYAHARA

Pratayahara is the act of consciously cutting off the mind from the senses. By doing this, the senses stop feeding the mind with stimulus and the yogi can bring consciousness to rest on the Self and not on external stimulation. This concept is stated in the Katha Upanishad and reads, "Know the self as a rider in a chariot, and the body, as simply the chariot. Know the intellect as the charioteer, and the mind, as simply the reins. The senses, they say, are the horses, and sense objects are the baths around them."[14]

6. DHARANA

Dharana is the first step towards a meditative state. In this initial phase, the yogi is working to focus their mind on a single point without distraction. Dharana is said to be achieved when one is able to master asana, pranayama, and pratayahara combined.

7. DHYANA

When concentration is able to be sustained without distraction, the yogi enters into a state of meditation. Imagine drops of water slowly dripping from your faucet. Each drop has its own form and is separate from the drop before it and the one after it. Think of each of these drops as individual thoughts. Now imagine you turned the faucet on until there was

---

[13] (Feuerstein G. , 1989)

[14] Katha Upanishad III 3-4

a steady stream of water. There is no longer a clear delineation of drops. They have merged together so any point along the stream looks exactly the same. This is a meditative state, where the last thought, the current thought and the next thought are all the same – a steady flow. This is achieved through time and practice.

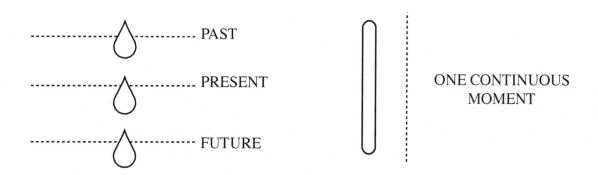

8. SAMADHI

Samadhi is the final limb but it is not the conclusion of one's practice. There are multiple states of Samadhi that peak with a state of Kivalya. Kivalya is a perpetual state of awareness. It is as to be in the world but not of the world.[15]

The state of Samadhi may be fleeting at first and must be cultivated over time. In samadhi one is said to have true understanding. In meditation, there is still an observed and an observer. The observed is able to remain constant but there is a subtle separation between the object and its observer. In Samadhi both the observed and the observer merge into one. There is no longer a separation and so there is no longer a duality of existence. This is why it has been described as a state of "oneness."

The limbs of yoga take time to cultivate and integrate into our lives. Inevitably there will be obstacles along the way. In Patanjali's Sutras there are nine obstacles listed.[16]

---

[15] (Desikachar, The Heart of Yoga: Developing A Personal Practice, 1999)

[16] *Yoga Sutra* 1.3

The nine obstacles are analogous to rocks or boulders set along our yoga path. They can slow, hinder or even stop the progression of our practice. Knowledge of these obstacles can help you recognize and overcome them when they occur.

1. **Illness:** Disease or sickness that robs us of focus or energy.

2. **Lethargy**: Dullness of mind, brought about by many factors including environmental.

3. **Doubt**: Questioning our decisions and motivations.

4. **Impatience**: Rushing through a step or activity. This is also linked to lack of foresight.

5. **Sloth**: Lack of enthusiasm and very little energy.

6. **Lack of detachment**: When the senses have the upper hand and think they are masters over the mind.

7. **Ignorance/arrogance:** Thinking we have reached the peak of the mountain so we act and speak as such. In reality we have a long way to go.

8. **Lack of perseverance:** Discouragement based on recognition of how far we have to go.

9. **Loss of confidence:** Developing feelings of insignificance as we progress along the path.

Thankfully the Sutras do not just list the obstacles, but they also offer practical techniques for overcoming them. In his book, The Heart of Yoga, Desikachar extracts these techniques from throughout the Sutras. They include finding a good teacher, exploring the senses (pratyahara), breathing techniques (pranayama), examination of spirit (dhyana), learning from role models, dream analysis, visualization techniques, mantras, and doing your best and surrender the rest to God (isvarapranidhana).

Additionally, the Sutras list four practices to help put the mind at ease.[17] These are friendliness towards those who are happy, compassion for those who are unhappy, Joy for those doing praiseworthy deeds, and indifference toward those in error. It has been pointed out that while indifference is a common translation, it is more accurately

---

[17] Yoga Sutras 1.33

described as 'a subtle and positive attitude', one of dispassionate but empathetic witnessing.[18]

---

[18] (Feuerstein G. , 1989)

The Seven Chakra System

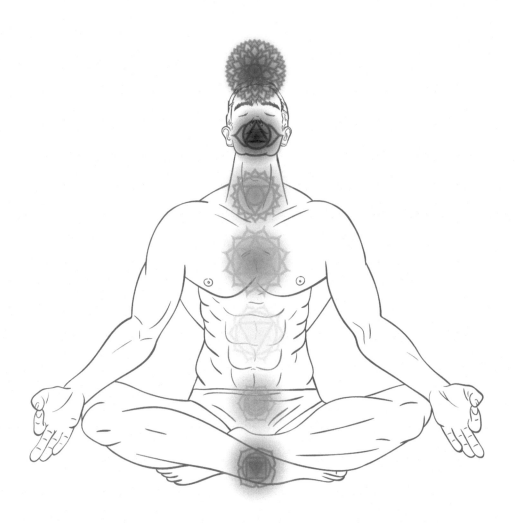

Sahasrara

Ajna

Vishuddha

Anahata

Manipura

Swadhisthana

Muladhara

1 Root (Muladhara)

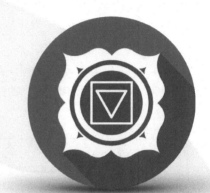

Area for Development

Foundation for emotional and mental health, learning to stand up for oneself

Body Connection

Bone, skeletal structure, base of spine, legs, feet, rectum, immune system

Physical Issues

Low back pain, osteoarthritis, immune disorders, varicose veins, sciatica

Emotional Issues

Depression, mental lethargy, personality disorders, obsessive-compulsive disorder, addictions

ASANA & EXERCISES

Sanskrit	Common		Exercises
Tadasana	Mountain		Reverse Hyper
Vrksasana	Tree		Body Squat
Utkatasana	Chair		Hip lifts
Trikonasana	Triangle		
Virasana	Hero		

NUTRITIONAL SUPPORT

Include	Limit
Blackberries, cherries, garlic, ginger, onions, pineapple, broccoli, chestnuts, clams, dandelion greens, flounder, hazelnuts, kale, kelp, oats, oysters, salmon, sea vegetables, sesame seeds, turnip greens	Sugar, ice cream, fried foods, peanuts, tobacco, alcohol, salt, citrus, tomatoes

2 Navel (Swadhisthana)

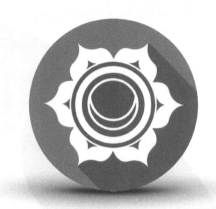

Area for Development	Challenging social conditioning, one-on-one relationships, sexuality, creativity and finance
Body Connection	Lower abdomen, sexual organs, large intestine, pelvis, appendix, bladder, hips
Physical Issues	Bladder and prostate problems, low back pain, arthritis, fibroids, sciatica
Emotional Issues	Unbalanced sex drive, emotional instability, isolation, fear of loss of control, fear of financial loss, abandonment issues, blame, guilt, power, control, ethics, honor

ASANA & EXERCISES

Sanskrit	Common
Alanasana	Crescent
Baddha Konasana	Bound Angle
Kapotasana	King Pigeon
Malasana	Garland
Gomukhasana	Cow Face
Padmasana	Lotus

Exercises
Leg Tuck
Pelvic Tilts
Piriformis Stretch
Lying Groin Stretch

NUTRITIONAL SUPPORT

Include	Limit
Asparagus, eggs, garlic, onions, green leafy vegetables, brown rice, avocados, fish, rye, fresh pineapple, flaxseed, apples, pears, green tea, milk thistle	Processed dairy, caffeine, citrus, paprika, salt, tobacco, sugar, (*peppers, *eggplant, *tomatoes, *white potatoes) *Night shade vegetables

56

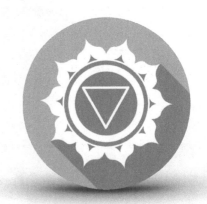

Area for Development	Self-confidence, draw and maintain self boundaries and personal code of honor
Body Connection	Abdomen, stomach, small intestine, liver, gallbladder, kidney, pancreas, adrenals, spleen, muscles
Physical Issues	Ulcers, intestinal problems, diabetes, indigestion, anorexia, bulimia, liver dysfunction, adrenal dysfunction
Emotional Issues	Oversensitive to criticism, low self esteem, need to be in control, fear of rejection, physical appearance anxieties, strength of character

ASANA & EXERCISES

Sanskrit	Common
Virabhadrasana II	Warrior II
Ardha Chandrasana	Half Moon
Natarajasana	Dancer
Parighasana	Beam
Vasisthasana	Side Plank
Apanasana	Knees to Chest
Navasana	Boat

Exercises
Elbow to Knee (table top)
Abdominal Crunches
Wood Chop
Fire Breath

NUTRITIONAL SUPPORT

Include	Limit
Dark green leafy vegetables, cabbage (fresh juice), avocados, bananas, potatoes, squash, yams, raw goats milk, kefir, chlorophyll, olive and safflower oil, salmon, tuna, brewers yeast, brown rice, legumes, dulse, kelp	Coffee, alcohol, fried foods, chocolate, soda, salt, sugar, refined carbohydrates, cows milk, NSAIDs* *Non Steroidal Anti-inflammatory Drugs

4 Heart (Anahata)

Area for Development	Forgiveness & compassion, mediation between body and spirit
Body Connection	Center of chest, heart, circulatory system, lungs, shoulders, arms and hands, ribs, diaphragm, thymus gland
Physical Issues	Shallow breathing, high blood pressure, heart disease, cancer, asthma, bronchial pneumonia, upper back, shoulder pain, breast issues
Emotional Issues	Fears of betrayal, co-dependency, hatred, bitterness, grief, anger, jealousy, fear of loneliness, inability to forgive

ASANA & EXERCISES

Sanskrit	Common
Matsyasana	Fish
Bhujangasana	Cobra
Ustrasana	Camel
Salabhasana	Locust
Adho Mukha Svanasana	Down-dog
Urdva Mukha Svanasana	Up-dog
Setu Banda Sarvangasana	Bridge

Exercises
Chaturanga Push-ups
Chi push/pull
Arm Circles
3 Part Breath

NUTRITIONAL SUPPORT

Include	Limit
Raw nuts (except peanuts), oatmeal, brown rice, garlic, onions, lemon (fresh juice), leafy green vegetables, herring, mackerel, turkey, trout	Ice cream, sugar, beans, broccoli, cauliflower, cabbage, processed dairy, coffee, black tea, alcohol, sugar, chocolate

5 Throat (Vishuddha)

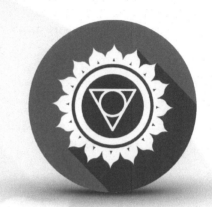

Area for Development	Personal expression, ability to release your will to divine guidance, faith – in fears or the divine?
Body Connection	Throat, thyroid, ears, mouth, teeth, gums, esophagus, parathyroid, hypothalamus, neck vertebrae
Physical Issues	Sore throat, mouth ulcers, gum difficulties, TMJ, scoliosis, laryngitis, swollen glands, thyroid problems
Emotional Issues	Perfectionism, inability to express emotions, blocked creativity, following your dream, using personal power to create, faith

ASANA & EXERCISES

Sanskrit	Common	Exercises
Uttanasana	Forward Fold	Neck Rotations
Prasarita Padottanasana	Standing Intense Spread-leg	Yes / No / Maybe
Parsvottanasana	Intense Side Stretch	Overhead Extensions
Paschimottanasana	Seated Forward Fold	Ujjayi Breath
Janu Sirsasana	Head-to-knee Pose	
Balasana	Crane	
Hanumanasana	Splits	

NUTRITIONAL SUPPORT

Include	Limit
Lemon, chamomile, honey, apricots, dates, egg yolks, parsley, prunes, raw seeds, raw milk, kelp, onion	Fluoride, sugar, white flour, processed food, alcohol, chewing gum, mouthwashes, tobacco

6 Third Eye (Ajna)

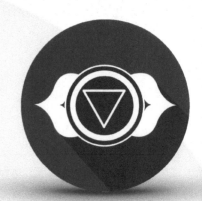

Area for Development

Intuition, emotional intelligence, reasoning. Using mental abilities and psychological skills to evaluate our beliefs and attitudes

Body Connection

Brain, nervous system, eyes, ears, nose, pineal gland, pituitary gland, base of skull

Physical Issues

Headaches, poor vision, neurological issues, hemorrhage , stroke, deafness, seizures

Emotional Issues

Hallucinations, learning difficulties, feelings of inadequacy, openness to the ideas of others, emotional intelligence

ASANA & EXERCISES

Sanskrit	Common
Parivrtta Trikonasana	Revolved Triangle
Parivrta Pasvakonasana	Revolved Side-angle
Bharadvajasana II	Bound Half-angle
Marichyasana I	Seated Spinal Twist
Jathara Parivartanasana	Reclining Spinal Twist

Exercises
Eye Rolling
Cow Face
Alternate Nostril Breath

NUTRITIONAL SUPPORT

Include	Limit
Water, carrots, collard greens, kale, mustard greens, spinach, blueberries, blackberries, cherries, cold pressed olive oil	Iced cream, iced beverages, salt, chewing gum, hot dogs, luncheon meats, alcohol, bananas, cheese, chicken, chocolate, herring, onions, peanut butter, pork, smoked fish, sour cream, vinegar

60

7 Crown (Sahasrara)

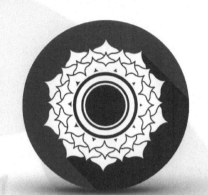

Area for Development

Selflessness, connection to our spiritual nature and allowing spirituality to become part of our physical lives

Body Connection

Upper skull, cerebral cortex, skin, muscular system, pineal gland

Physical Issues

Sensitivity to pollutants & light, chronic exhaustion, epilepsy, Alzheimer's

Emotional Issues

Spirituality and devotion, depression, confusion, obsessive thinking, courage, ethics, humanitarianism

ASANA & EXERCISES

Sanskrit	Common
Garudasana	Eagle
Virabhadrasana III	Warrior III
Bakasana	Crow / Crane
Sarvangasana	Shoulder Stand
Sirsasana	Headstand
Halasana	Plow

Exercises
Seated Meditation
Mantra's
Supine Surrender

NUTRITIONAL SUPPORT

Include	Limit
*Balanced diet in accordance with your Metabolic Type™. Have hair tissue mineral analysis to rule out the presence of heavy metals.	Alcohol, tobacco, tap water, fried and processed foods

61

Understanding the Chakra System

"It is not enough to merely understand without action or to merely move energy without understanding. It is the integration of these two currents that creates the changes we seek in our lives." – Anodea Judith

Prana is the subtle life force energy that fills and surrounds all things. Subtle energy is conscious while gross energy is not.[19] Prana travels the subtle body through nadis. Think of nadis like a hose and prana like the water. These nadis converge in larger numbers at seven power centers in your body, called chakras. The word chakra means "disk" or "wheel of light." You will also sometimes see it written as cakra.

The state of each chakra is reflected in your physical, psychological, emotional and spiritual well-being. A healthy, open, balanced chakra spins in a clockwise motion (viewed looking at an individual). When chakra energy is blocked, misdirected, or stagnant, emotional and physical illness can arise. Introspection, prayer, visualization, pranayama, and the willingness to change our outlook are essential to working with the subtle body.

It is important to realize that chakras respond to our constructive attention. If we long for the will to live a more refined and enlightened life, and if we exercise that will, all of these centers increase their power and ability.

Are Chakras Real?
The answer to that question may depend on our definition of "real." Chakras are centers of spiritual energy. As the metaphysical teacher and clairvoyant Barbara Martin puts it, "[Chakras] are receiving and transmitting stations for spiritual energy flowing in and out of the aura."[20] Spiritual energy is not physical energy and so it cannot be measured by physical tools.

---

[20] (Moraitis, 2006)

How then do we know of their existence? The Hindus, Tibetans, Chinese, Incans, Hebrews, Tsalagi (Cherokee) Native Americans, Egyptians, and Africans historically all had maps of an energy anatomy connected to the human body.[21] While each is not exactly the same, they are strikingly similar in many ways. Aside from the fact that these major cultures living thousands of miles apart from one another came to report very similar systems, we also have the testimony of the clairvoyants, and mystics who can see the subtle energy fields of the aura and chakras.[22]

Chakra Summaries
Muladhara (root)

The first chakra is located at the base of the spine near the perineum or cervix. It relates to our survival and self-preservation as well as the dormant inner kundalini power. In Tantric yoga this is the location of Shakti, the divine feminine energy.

Svadishthana (dwelling place of the self)

The second chakra is located in the lower abdomen behind the genitals and sacrum. It relates to sexuality emotions, our ability to create and nurture as well as to love. This chakra also relates to the collective unconscious.

Manipura (lustrous gem)

The third chakra is located behind the navel, corresponding to the solar plexus. It relates to our willpower, creative energy, digestion, imagination and self-definition.

Anahata (unstruck or unbroken)

---

[21] (Dale, 2009)

[22] I am not suggesting that one should take the testimony of anyone claiming to see chakras as truth. However there have been studies testing some people's abilities to recognize disease in the body through their clairvoyance and matching it up against medical exams by doctors. The accuracy of some was incredibly high.

The fourth chakra is located in the heart area. It relates to love, relationships, compassion, and self-acceptance. It is connected to our social identity as we learn to love our self as well as to love others.

Vishuddha (purification)

The fifth chakra is located at the throat. It relates to communication and self-expression; our ability to be able to speak and be heard. It also relates to our creative identity and spiritual drive.

Ajna (to perceive and to know)

The sixth chakra is located near the brow just above and between the eyes. This chakra is sometimes referred to as the third eye. It relates to our intuition, imagination, intelligence and clarity.

Sahasrara (thousand fold or thousand-petaled lotus)

The seventh chakra is located just above the top of the head. It relates to the governing of our cerebral cortex, pure awareness and self-knowledge. Sahasrara is considered to be beyond the senses and sense organs, and most closely related to our spiritual connection.

The Philosophy of Pranayama

Prana, as defined earlier, is subtle energy. It is the equivalent to the Chinese Chi and the Japanese Ki respectively. The concept of subtle energy is one that has been part of many cultures throughout history, and the discipline of yoga is no exception. In yoga philosophy pranic energy flows through an intricate superhighway of channels called nadis. The exact number of nadis in the body is hard to ascertain because they appear to change throughout yoga's history and are dependent upon the authority at the time.

Regardless, three major channels stay consistent throughout. They are Sushumna, the center channel which runs the length of the spinal cord; Ida and Pingala.

Ida starts on the left side of the pelvis at the root chakra and weaves back and forth up the spine intersecting at each chakra center until it reaches the third eye. From there it turns back down and ends at the left nasal passageway.

Pingala starts on the right side of the pelvis and continues in the same manner as Ida but on the opposite side, ending at the right nasal passageway. Ida is the channel for more yin, feminine energy, while Pingala is the channel for more yang masculine energy. In Tantric philosophy Shakti energy (divine feminine) lives at the root chakra, while Shiva energy (divine masculine) lives at the crown chakra. Shiva and Shakti are like to sides of the same coin. The process of Kundalini rising is the process of bringing pranic energy from Shakti up to Shiva, completing the totality of the divine by uniting them. This movement of energy is often pictured as two snakes weaving up a staff. They cross at five locations along the way.[23]

Collectively prana, nadis, and chakras make up much of the anatomy of our subtle body. In yoga, the subtle body is referred to as pranamaya Kosa. Kosas are sheaths or layers of the self. Imagine the five Kosas like Russian dolls, one layered inside another from the outer surface to the core of the Self.

Our breath has a powerful effect on pranic energy and how it flows. Prana is described as something that flows continuously from deep within. A state of disease, lethargy, frustration, or feeling stuck, is an expression of too much prana outside the body. The more peaceful and balanced we feel, the less dispersed our prana is outside the body. If the prana does not have room to flow freely within the body, then something must be blocking it. These blocks are the "trash" which the breath helps to release. Breathing enables us to open ourselves to receive more prana within while allowing it to flow freely at the same time.

Inhale (Puraka)	Exhale (Rechaka)	Pause x2 (Kumbhaka)
warming	cooling	neutral
openness	defining boundaries	vulnerability
motion	grounding	stillness
spaciousness	centeredness	potential
light	dark	balanced

---

[23] (Desikachar, The Heart of Yoga: Developing A Personal Practice, 1999)

Since our breathing has a direct influence on our mind, we use pranayama-breathing exercises to steady the mind, draw in more prana and balance the energies of the body.[24]

When we breathe, we move the five types of vital energy called prana-vayus. They are Prana, Apana, Samana, Adana, and Vyana. Prana-vayu runs in the thoracic region and controls breathing. Apana moves in the lower belly and controls elimination. Samana aides in digestion and maintaining balance in the abdominal organs. Adana controls the vocal chords and food and air intake. Vyana travels through the entire body moving the energy from food and breath through the blood.

On an inhale breath Prana-vayu is activated lifting the panic energy while on the exhale Apana-vayu is activated lowering the pranic energy.

The parts of breath

The breath itself has four parts to it. The inhale is characterized as lifting Prana-vayu. Inhales create more space and openness. This space is easy to experience with a seated twist. You can feel the rib cage attempt to expand out and open, lifting the torso. The exhale in contrast allows us space to ground down and deepen the twist. The exhale is characterized as engaging Apana-vayu, the downward flowing energy. It is more grounding and centering. Exhales bring us back to our core. There are two pauses to the breath, one at the top of the inhale and one at the bottom of the exhale. The pause is neutral and characterized as the point of potentiality. There are infinite possibilities at the point of complete stillness. A holding the breath at the bottom of an exhale can give us a feeling of vulnerability as well.

Beginning your practice

The techniques described below are sometimes referred to as "soft pranayama." This is a term to describe basic techniques which are thought to be safe for the average person. Of course, you should always practice with awareness and stop at any sign of discomfort. If you have any question about whether or not pranayama is safe, you should consult with

---

[24] Desikachar, The Heart of Yoga, Developing A Personal Practice, 1999

your doctor. It is not necessary to sit for hours of pranayama to begin to experience the benefits. In fact, for most people, it is probably unrealistic to do this. Instead, keep the practice short, 3-25 minutes to begin, and consistent. Consistency, like with yogasana, is the key.

Building Up

Abdominal Breathing:

Lie down on your back in Corpse Pose with your hands on your abdomen. Begin to draw awareness to the breath observing its quality and quantity. Draw the attention of the mind down to the abdomen. Begin to control the breath by breathing deep into the abdomen allowing it to expand up towards the sky on the inhale and sink down to the earth on the exhale. Continue to breathe this way for 3-5 minutes.

This type of breath creates a relaxation response in the body by stimulating a neurological sensor called the baroreceptor, located on the wall of the descending aorta. The baroreceptor is a mechanoreceptor that senses changes in blood pressure and heart rate. Baroreceptor activation stimulates the hypothalamus in the brain to lower heart rate and blood pressure.

Wave Breathing (3-part breath):

Find either a comfortable seated or lying position. Inhale and allow the collar bones to expand first, followed by the sternum, and finally the abdomen. With your exhale, reverse the motion from the abdomen, to the sternum, and finally the upper chest. Practice creating an evenness of motion in all three parts of the breath. Try to balance the length of inhalation and exhalation with one another.

With practice, your breath will begin to slow to 8 to 10 breaths per minute rather than the average 12 to 15. This technique helps to strengthen and coordinate the muscles of respiration giving you greater conscious control over them. This control is beneficial as you continue with your pranayama practice.

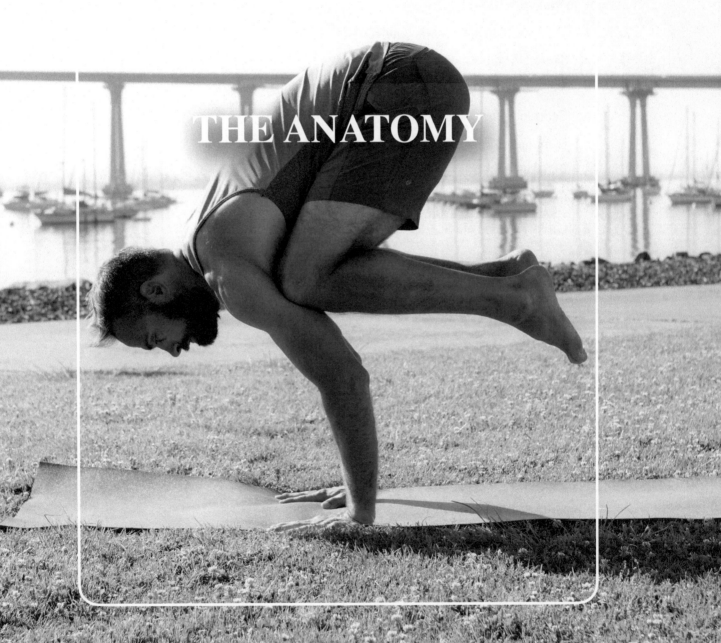

THE ANATOMY

THE ANATOMY

What You Need to Know and What You Don't

I have been leading yoga trainings, workshops and classes for close to ten years now. Throughout that time, I've come to one very basic but profound understanding. KEEP IT SIMPLE. The human body is a vastly complex organism with multiple systems working independently and interdependently. Just think about the eleven major systems working right now in your body:

1. Muscular (muscle fibers, connective tissue)
2. Skeletal (bones, connective tissue)
3. Nervous (Brain, spinal cord, peripheral nerves
4. Endocrine (hormone)
5. Lymphatic (immune)
6. Reproductive (testicles, ovaries, uterus etc.)
7. Integumentary (skin)
8. Urinary (kidneys, bladder, urethra)
9. Digestive (small and large intestine, gallbladder, pancreas, liver, stomach)
10. Cardiovascular (heart, veins, arteries, blood)
11. Respiratory (lungs, esophagus, larynx, mouth, nose, muscles)

Each one of these systems carries out multiple tasks and coordinates with multiple other systems to create an internal balance regardless of the always changing outside stimulus.

So exactly how much anatomy does a yoga student, or teacher for that matter, need to know? It's a great question. My answer is this. One, you should have a basic understanding of the systems that relate to the practice of yoga. Two, you should keep it simple to avoid paralysis through analysis. Remember that yoga is a practice. It needs to be engaged with and explored through action. Yoga does not live in the pages of a book, it lives in you. I've tried to keep the anatomy and physiology to a level that is easily digestible (no pun intended), and that will be useful to you in your practice. Throughout this book I have included anatomical information as they related to the practice being discussed. This is not solely an anatomy book. It is a yoga book.

That being said, some people truly enjoy learning about the detailed workings of the human body. If you are one of those people there are some wonderful texts on the subject, including work by Mel Robin, David Coulter, Ray Long and David Keil to name a few.

Your depth of study in anatomy, will largely depend upon your intention with yoga. For those who are interested in becoming teachers I have included below "key terms" that you will see in many anatomy books. Knowing these terms will help you in your studies.

KEY TERMS

Anatomy: The branch of science concerned with the bodily structure of humans. . . especially as revealed by the dissection and the separation of its parts.

Physiology: The way in which a living organism or bodily part functions.

Kinesiology: The study of the mechanics of body movement.

Flexibility: The quality of bending easily without breaking.

Stretch: (of something soft or elastic) Being capable of being made wider or longer without tearing or breaking.

Isometric: Muscular action in which tension is developed without contraction of the muscle.

Isotonic: Taking place with normal contraction.

Muscle: A band or bundle of fibrous tissue in a human or animal body that has the ability to contract, producing movement in or maintaining the position of parts of the body.

Connective Tissue: Tissue that connects, supports, binds, or separates other tissues or organs, typically having relatively few cells embedded in an amorphous matrix often with collagen or other fibers, and including cartilaginous, fatty, and elastic tissues.

Fascia: A thin sheath of fibrous tissue enclosing a muscle or other organ.

Ligament: A short band of tough, flexible, fibrous connective tissue that connects two bones or cartilages or holds together a joint.

Tendon: A flexible but inelastic cord of strong fibrous collagen tissue attaching a muscle to a bone.

The kinetic chain: All human movement occurs via the Kinetic chain. This is the interconnectedness of three systems: the muscular, skeletal and nervous.

Planes of Movement

The body moves through a variety of planes. Each one has associated movement patterns. The planes of movement are sagittal, coronal, and transverse. The chart below shows the associated movement patterns in more detail.

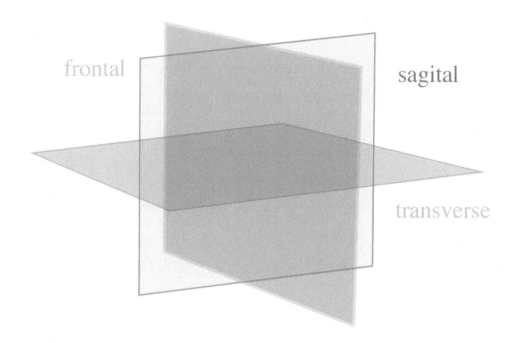

In the proper sequencing of a yogasana class, we move the spine and limbs through all planes of motion.

- **Coronal -** Adduction/Abduction
- **Sagittal -** Flexion/Extension
- **Transverse -** Internal Rotation / External Rotation

Anatomic Locations

- Anterior – Towards the front
- Posterior – Towards the back

- Superior - Above
- Inferior - Below
- Medial – Towards the midline
- Lateral – Away from the midline

Your Practice, Your Body

I once sat in on a workshop delivered by Max Payne, the Director of the Yoga Therapy program at Loyola Marymount University. The workshop gave me many new useful tools for teaching, but there was one thing in particular that stood out to me, and I say it frequently in my classes: You should never try to jam your body to fit a cookie cutter image of a posture. Instead, you should adjust the posture to fit your body.

In yoga philosophy, the physical world is continuously changing. Our bodies are no exception to this rule. We have to consider all of our converging histories and how they have made us who we are today when we step on our mats. Our histories need to include our injuries, mental states, natural physical abilities and anatomy.[25]

When we do this, it becomes evident that the "by the book description" is good, but we are not in a book, we are alive, dynamic organisms and we need to honor this. We can do this by making the pose fit our own body rather than trying to fit our body into the pose.

In this next section, we will talk about some of the basic principles of alignment and how to customize our practice so that it is always a reflection of who we are for that day and that practice only. Doing this will not only make your practice safer, but it will also make the practice more enjoyable, giving you the confidence to take any class, anywhere, at any time.

Basic Principles of Alignment

Alignment principles are established from a static upright standing position. The body's skeleton is held together by connective tissues and muscles. The tension of muscle fibers pulls on the bones and can pull the body out of correct alignment.

---

[25] (Keil D. , 2014)

What is correct alignment? Webster Dictionary defines alignment as "being in the correct or appropriate positions." In terms of yoga, correct alignment is about establishing the correct positions of the bones, which then creates correct positions in the joints. If the joint is not in the appropriate position when the body moves, or if it is not able to remain in its appropriate position through its range of motion, it can lead to pain or injury. There are specific landmark cues we use to establish whether or not a person's body is in correct alignment. These landmarks are called kinetic checkpoints. They are: ankles, knees, hips, spine, shoulders and head.

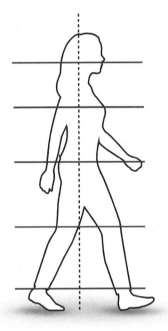

When two bones use the maximum surface area available to fit together correctly, the joint is in a state of congruency. If a joint becomes incongruent (especially in load bearing joints), then the pressure is not evenly distributed within the joint and the area that holds the most pressure could be harmed.

Human evolution: from sea star to upright walking in a 18 months

We as humans mimic evolution through our gestation from single celled organisms to human babies. Beyond that I've taken the three major systems of the kinetic chain (skeletal, muscular and nervous) and summarized them with details on any aspects that relate to our asana practice.

Our sense of movement begins in utero with the development of the vestibular system. These receptors in the inner ear are responsible for keeping us balanced in a field of gravity after birth, but even before that they are communicating information on position within the womb. This is why babies like to be bounced and rocked. The movement replicates that which was felt by the vestibular system before birth. Additionally, proprioceptive and kinesthetic nerves in the bones, joints, muscles, fascia and ligaments communicate information about touch pressure, rhythm, and vibration teaching us about our environment through our movement.[26]

After birth, we develop through a series of movement patterns. At first, we effectively have six limbs: head, arms, legs and tail. Our movement occurs from what is called a navel radiation pattern. The navel is the center of axis from which movement radiates out. The nerves of the limbs have not yet myelinated (developed a protective sheath around the nerve that amplifies and directs its signals to skeletal muscles) and so they flail around wildly. Occasionally all four limbs will rapidly extend out, startling the newborn. This is the navel radiation pattern in action.

The head and tail are used to wiggle around on our backs. This head movement is further strengthened by the sucking pattern. A newborn will go to a mother's breast almost immediately after birth to nurse.

Once a baby can roll over, its next instinct is to lift its head and begin a push pattern, initiating the child's inner awareness of weight, gravity, balance and movement. Pressing away from the earth is a powerful movement of independence and autonomy as an individual. Following the push pattern is a reach and pull pattern. Here the child starts to develop a curiosity about the world. With the head lifted and the development of the ears and eyes, the reach and pull movements develop as a way to explore.[27]

From here the movements will build upon one and another until the child moves towards an upright position. This involves a *squat* position and finally a *gate*. Using the hands as a base of support against a fixed object a child will *push* with their legs as they reach and *pull* with their arms. The vestibular system continues to develop to establish and understanding of the body in space against the force of gravity. Once steady on their feet, walking will begin. This requires a static postural balance to then be integrated into dynamic movement.

In order to maintain an upright position, the body needs to have developed both righting and equilibrium reflexes. The majority of righting reflexes are built into our nervous system by the age three. Righting reflexes keep the head in a normal position and

---

[26] (Hartley, 1995)

[27] (Hartley, 1995)

adjust the body to a normal position. They tend to be dominant when moving across a fixed or stable surface. In contrast, equilibrium reflexes do the same but are more dominant when the surface below us moves.[28] These reflexes develop progressively with time.

From a developmental standpoint, a majority of the primal or functional movement patterns are present from the very beginning of our lives. They have been built in through hundreds of thousands, if not millions, of years. It is vital to maintain these functional movement patterns in order to move our bodies in the optimal way, and avoid injury.

Physical stress occurs every day of your life. As you move throughout your day you experience the stress of gravity against your body. Without it the muscles, bones ligaments and tendons would atrophy, and the body would begin to break down. This is why astronauts working in zero gravity conditions have special exercise equipment to keep their body fit for life under earth's gravity. If you've ever broken a bone you've experienced this weakening first hand (no pun intended). Take for example a broken arm. The arm would usually be placed within a cast for four to six weeks. When the cast is removed, you can notice a clear difference between the limb of the broken arm and the limb of the other. Without the stress of daily use the muscles of the casted arm began to atrophy and break down.

Physical stress can be acute or chronic. An acute stress would be considered something like a broken bone or sprained ankle. An outside force has caused the body physical injury (stress) from which it needs to heal. Chronic physical stress can be skeletal and muscular imbalances, inadequate rest or over training. Another form of physical stress is diet.

If the body is imbalanced from the standpoint of the skeletal and muscular system, it will be constantly allocating energy to attempt to correct these imbalances. Rounded shoulders, and weak core musculature can lead to an inverted breathing pattern known as upper chest breathing. This type of breathing stimulates the sympathetic nervous system

---

[28] (Chek, 2011)

by taking short shallow breaths, throwing the rest of the body into a subtle but chronic stressed state.

Poor posture and repetitive movements create dysfunction in the kinetic chain. The body initiates a repair process called the cumulative injury cycle.[29] If not interrupted by correcting postural imbalances, the cycle continues, altering neuromuscular control and causing connective tissue adhesions. You may have felt these adhesions or had them pointed out to you by a massage therapist as "knots" in the muscles. It is not actually a knot in the muscle, but in the connective tissue that surrounds the muscle. Our connective tissue is directly connected to pain receptors in the brain. Creating flexibility and strength in our connective tissue coupled using breath and asana has been shown to release endorphins and calm pain receptors in the brain. A well sequenced yoga class helps to stretch overactive muscles and strengthen underactive ones, putting the body back into correct postural alignment and breaking the cumulative injury cycle.

The Kinetic Chain

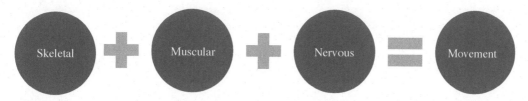

Biomechanics: The central and peripheral nervous systems communicate with skeletal muscles via nerve pathways. These pathways assess and interpret both the internal and external environment to determine the correct action (movement). This can be demonstrated in the reflex that takes place when you jump from a high surface. Your body activates the correct muscles in the correct way to stabilize you so you don't fall over. This takes very little conscious thought on your part.

---

[29] (Michael A. Clark, 2008)

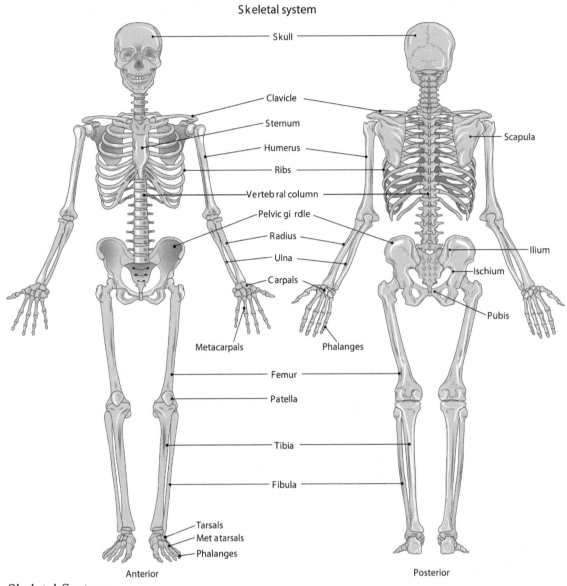

Skeletal system

Skull

Clavicle

Sternum

Humerus

Ribs

Vertebral column

Pelvic girdle

Radius

Ulna

Carpals

Metacarpals

Phalanges

Femur

Patella

Tibia

Fibula

Tarsals

Metatarsals

Phalanges

Scapula

Ilium

Ischium

Pubis

Anterior

Posterior

Skeletal System

Overview

Our skeleton is made up of our bones. Bone is actually living tissue that has the ability to grow and heal from injury and stress. Applying the correct amount of stress through exercise like asana helps to keep our bones and joints strong and healthy into the later years of our lives.

Bones are the framework that we use to give shape to asana. They are made up of calcium, phosphorus, sodium, and other minerals, as well as the protein collagen. Bones give stability and protection to the body through their various structures. Bones come in a variety of different shapes depending upon their location and ultimately their function. Here is a list of the common shapes of bones, their function and examples.

- Long bones - Provide leverage (femur, tibia, humerus)
- Short bones - Weight bearing with no hollow cavity (carpal and tarsal bones)
- Flat bones - Provide protection and places for broad muscles to attach (cranial bones, scapulae, ribs, pelvis)
- Irregular bones- Have two or more different shapes (vertebrae)

The skeleton is subdivided into two different categories, the axial and appendicular. The axial skeleton is composed of the skull, spinal column, rib cage, and pelvic girdle. It is the axis around which yoga poses revolve. The appendicular skeleton is composed of the multiple bones of the arms and the legs. It connects us to each other and the earth. The arms and legs are also the levers we use to move the axial skeleton.

The Appendicular and Axial Skeleton
The skeleton is divided into two sections. The Axial Skelton, which is comprised of the skull, spinal cord and pelvic girdle, and the Appendicular Skeleton, which is composed of the arms and legs. In yogasana, we use our appendicular skeleton to move our axial skeleton. A simple example of this is to consider the way that the arms can deepen the twist in the spine when we move into a Crescent Twisted Pose.

The Spine
The Spine is composed of five different sections. It has the very important function of protecting our spinal cord which runs through each one of the vertebrae as mentioned when discussing "Maintaining Strength in Your Core."

The coccyx is located at the base of the spine and is composed of four fused vertebrae.

The sacrum is located above the coccyx. It is composed of five vertebrae that fuse in our youth. It is located between the ilium bones. The joint where the sacrum and the illium meet is called the sacroiliac joint. This joint has limited mobility and moves primarily forward and backward (nutation and counter nutation). I explain in earlier sections the significance of protecting the SA joint in certain twisting poses.

Above the sacrum is the lumbar spine. It is composed of five vertebrae. The lumbar section of the spine has a lordotic curve which makes this section of the spine more conducive to backbending. However, as explained in earlier sections, we need to use caution in asana in order to protect this area of our spine. The lumbar spine is also one of the most common places for people to experience injuries like a bulging or slipped disk.

HUMAN VERTEBRAL COLUMN

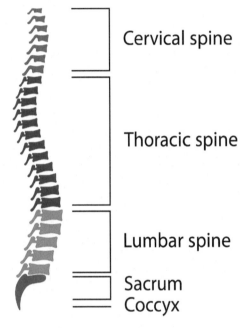

Cervical spine

Thoracic spine

Lumbar spine

Sacrum
Coccyx

Above the lumbar spine is the thoracic spine. It is composed of 12 vertebrae arranged in a kyphotic curve, which makes this section of the spine more conducive to forward folds. It is this section of the spine that our ribs connect to.

Above the thoracic spine is the cervical spine. It is composed of seven vertebrae arranged in a lordotic curve. The first and second vertebrae of the cervical spine are called the atlas and the axis. These vertebrae have a slightly different shape. The atlas has a pronounced hump that lifts up into the center ring of the atlas allowing for a greater range of motion for the head. The cervical vertebrae are arranged in a way that anatomically is not conducive to neck rolling, despite the very common practice of doing this in a yoga class. This is covered in greater depth in the earlier section entitled "The Five Things You're Doing that Cause Injury."

A tip for remembering the number of vertebrae (excluding the sacrum and coccyx) is to think about breakfast, lunch, dinner.

Section of Spine	Number of Vertebra	Curve	Remember
Cervical	7	Lordosis	Breakfast 7 am
Thoracic	12	Kyphosis	Lunch 12 pm
Lumbar	5	Lordosis	Dinner 5 pm
		Total	24*

* your spine works for you 24 hours a day

The Spine has curves for a reason, protect them
When the human fetus is growing in utero, the spine develops a primary curve. This primary curve is a "C" shape that we can easily picture when imagining a baby curled up in the fetal position.

One of the first movements a newborn baby has after its great adventure from the inside to the outside world is to get into a position to nurse. Once it has established a latch with the mother, it begins to suck. This process is not only essential for feeding, it is also an important engagement of the muscles in the jaw, head, and neck. These muscles will continue to strengthen for the next few months until a baby learns how to roll over and lift its head.

When a baby begins to lift its head, it begins to develop the cervical (neck) curve in its spine. This curve will continue to develop as the muscles of the core, arms, legs and back strengthen, eventually leading to the baby getting up onto all fours.

Once on all fours, the curve of the lumbar spine develops (low back). Gravity pulls the hips forward and the belly down encouraging the development of the lumbar curve.

At about a year old the baby will begin to test the ability to get onto two feet, eventually standing and walking for the rest of its life in the bipedal position. The curves that developed in this first year are important to the spine's overall strength and functionality. As Mel Robin has pointed out, "Were the spine to grow into a rigid, straight rod, then walking would be difficult, for the jolt of every footstep would be transmitted directly to the brain."[30]

---

[30] (Robin, 2009)

The curves of the spine allow the spine to act more like a spring, absorbing the weight of gravity through the process of running, walking, squatting, pushing, lunging and more.

Types of Joints

A joint is created anywhere two bones come together. Different shapes of bones coming together create different types of joints. The type of joint also defines the way that it moves. Here is a list of the major classifications of joint types.

- Hinge – elbows and knees
- Ball and Socket – shoulders and hips
- Gliding – hands and feet
- Saddle – base of the thumb
- Condyloid - fingers
- Pivot – radius and ulna of the arms and the tibia and fibula of the legs

3 key components of Joints

While a joint is defined as the point where two bones come together, there are additional components that make up the anatomy of a joint.

1. Bone: Long, short, flat, etc.
2. Soft tissue: Ligaments, cartilage, meniscus, labrum, etc.
3. Muscles: Muscle and tendon

Of these various types the most significant for our asana practice are the hinge, and ball and socket joints.

Hinge joints are located at the elbows and knees. They primarily move through flexion and extension. The knee however does allow for slight rotation after 10° of flexion.[31] This rotation is what makes lotus pose possible for many. Hyperextension of hinge joints is common and should be avoided. If you notice that your knees or elbows hyperextend (extend past 180° of extension) you should use slight muscular engagement to bring the joint back to congruency.

---

[31] (Keil K. , 2014)

Joint congruency is when the articular surfaces of a joint fit together perfectly, maximizing the surface area of the bones coming together to create that joint.[32] It's important to keep joints as congruent as possible especially when they are weight bearing because if you don't, it adds much more pressure to a smaller section of the joint. Think of a bed of nails. If you were to lie on a bed of 1,000 nails your body weight would be spread out over each nail you touched, putting only a little weight on each nail. If however, you were to lie on a bed of only four nails, there would be quite a bit more weight on each nail. When a joint is congruent the force on the joint is spread out evenly across a wider surface area. If it is not congruent, more force is placed on a smaller surface area which could cause injury.

Ball and socket joints are located at the hips and shoulders. The hip joint is a much deeper socket compared to the shoulder join since it has to hold the weight of the upper body. A good rule to remember is *if a joint has a wider range of motion it is less stable, if it has a limited range of motion it is more stable.* The shoulder joint is a much shallower socket and is held in place more by the muscular and connective tissue surrounding it. This provides for a wider range of motion but limited stability. For this reason we have to be particularly careful with how we align our arms in certain yoga poses. It's best to stack the long axis of the bones. For example in side plank pose (Vasisthasana), the wrist is directly under the radius and ulna which are directly under the humerus with the shoulder at the top.

The shoulders, elbows, hips, and knees are synovial joints. synovial joints are wrapped in dense irregular connective tissue to create the joint capsule. Within the joint capsule is synovial fluid which lubricates the joint. The more a synovial joint is used the less viscous the synovial fluid is, which facilitates easy movement. Cartilage on the end of a bone provides a smooth slippery surface for the bones to slide over one and other without abrasion. The labrum of the hips and meniscus of the knees provide cushion and help maintain integrity in the joints.

---

[32] (Long MD, FRCSC, 2006)

Structure of Skeletal Muscle

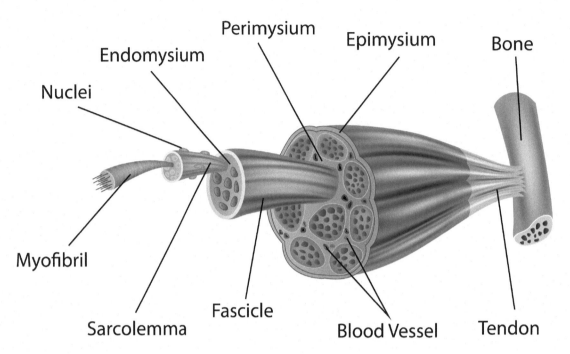

Moving the body regularly with functional integrated patterns like yogasana help to keep the joints healthy and the skeleton in proper alignment. That being said, bones don't move themselves, they have to be moved. That happens through the contract release patterns of the muscles.

Muscular System

Muscles move the body via the signals from the nervous system. Afferent nerves in the body gather information from the outside world (sense) and communicate it back to the brain. Efferent nerves then send a signal back to the correct muscles to take action. For example if you put your hand on a hot pan on the stovetop. Very quickly your body will sense the heat and pull your hand away from the hot surface.

A muscle is composed of various groupings of tissues and fibers. Fibers are grouped into fascicles which are grouped into bundles. Muscles are attached to bones by tendons at the origin and insertion points. Muscle fibers contract in response to afferent nerve stimuli. Muscles exist in either a contracted, relaxed or stretched state.

Muscles that cross only one joint are classified as monoarticular. When these muscles contract they primarily move only one joint. An example of this are the iliacus muscles located along the inner side of the hip (ilium bone). Muscles that cross more than one joint are classified as polyarticular. When these muscles contract they can move multiple joints. An example of this would be the psoas. The psoas originates at the 1st-4th lumbar vertebra crossing multiple vertebra before crossing the hip joint and inserting at the greater trochanter of the femur.

According to the 2016 Yoga In America study conducted by Yoga Alliance and Yoga Journal, one of the top three reasons people begin yoga is to improve their flexibility. Muscles can become tight from repetitive movement or from lack of use. Stretching a muscle, as is done in many yoga poses, increases its flexibility.

Physiology of Stretch

Different stretch techniques can be applied in different situations to stretch a muscle. These techniques are based on an understanding of how the nervous system affects the muscular system. Listed below are three physiological responses in the body that are the basis for the stretch techniques used by yoga teachers, physical therapists and other body workers.

1. **Muscle spindle relaxation response**:   Within the belly of each muscle are proprioceptors called muscle spindles. These receptors communicate to the brain the length tension relationship within a muscle. They help us to control our movements so a forward fold doesn't look like someone dropping the strings of a puppet. When we hold a stretch for 30-60 seconds the muscle spindles slow down their signaling to the brain. Without a clear image of the length tension relationship the muscle can relax further and allow us to stretch deeper.

2. **Reciprocal inhibition**:   The biceps muscles flex the arm and the triceps muscles extend the arm. If I were to hold my arm out by my side fully extended with my palm

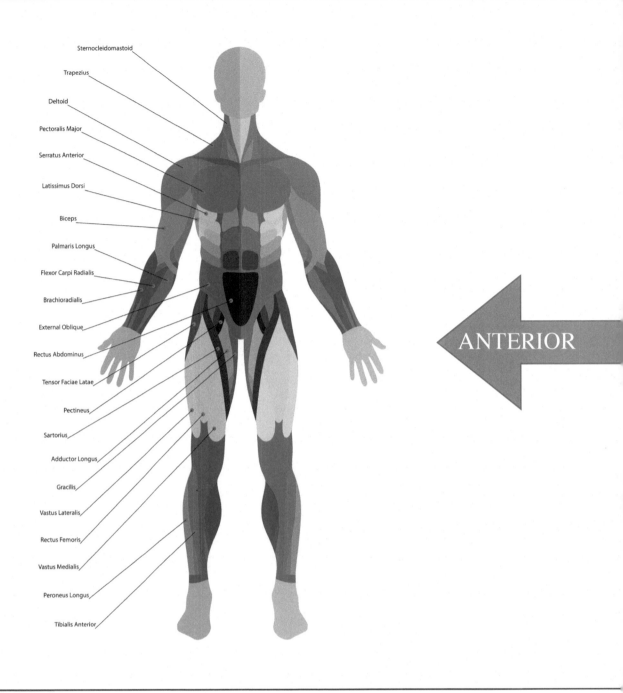

Sternocleidomastoid

Trapezius

Deltoid

Pectoralis Major

Serratus Anterior

Latissimus Dorsi

Biceps

Palmaris Longus

Flexor Carpi Radialis

Brachioradialis

External Oblique

Rectus Abdominus

Tensor Faciae Latae

Pectineus

Sartorius

Adductor Longus

Gracilis

Vastus Lateralis

Rectus Femoris

Vastus Medialis

Peroneus Longus

Tibialis Anterior

ANTERIOR

up, and then slowly flex my elbow, my biceps would be contracting to pull the forearm and create the bend. If on the opposite side of my arm, my triceps were to contract at the same time they would be working opposite my biceps, halting the movement of flexion. Reciprocal inhibition is a nervous system loop: when one muscle is trying to contact, its opposite muscle needs to relax. The technical terms are agonist and antagonist. The agonist muscle is the one that is trying to contract. In the above example this is the biceps. The antagonist muscles are then the triceps. With reciprocal inhibition we trick the body into relaxing the muscle we want to stretch by contracting its opposite.

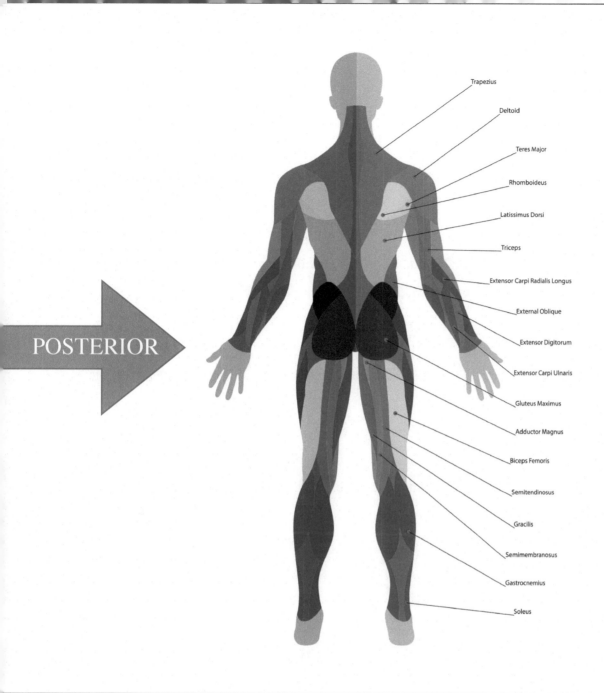

POSTERIOR

Trapezius
Deltoid
Teres Major
Rhomboideus
Latissimus Dorsi
Triceps
Extensor Carpi Radialis Longus
External Oblique
Extensor Digitorum
Extensor Carpi Ulnaris
Gluteus Maximus
Adductor Magnus
Biceps Femoris
Semitendinosus
Gracilis
Semimembranosus
Gastrocnemius
Soleus

For example, If I am in a standing forward fold, I am stretching (among other things) my hamstrings on the backs of my upper legs. If I were to use reciprocal inhibition, I would contract my quadriceps on the upper front of my legs. This would relax my hamstrings and once it did this I could stretch deeper into the pose.

3. **Golgi tendon organ**: The golgi tendon organ is a proprioceptor that is located at the musculotendinous junction (point where the muscle meets the tendon). Its job is to sense the tension at this point to insure that there is not too much strain which could

lead to injury. Using a facilitated stretch technique explained below we can trick the golgi tendon organ into giving us more space to stretch into the desired muscle.

Four methods for stretching muscles

Once the physiology of stretching is understood, specific stretch techniques can be implemented throughout our practice to improve flexibility and range of motion in joints. Below are four stretch techniques. I recommend only three of them. .

1. **Ballistic stretching**: Ballistic stretching uses jumping or bouncing type actions to stretch targeted muscles. Some studies show that this can create micro tears in the muscle. It's my opinion that this type of stretching should be avoided. Ballistic stretching is sometimes confused with dynamic stretching but they are not the same thing. Dynamic stretching uses steady deliberate movements that follow the breath. Suryanamaskara A is a great example. Each breath has an associated movement (stretch) but there is no bouncing (quick repetitive contract / release) movements.

2. **Passive stretching:** This stretch technique uses body weight and gravity to hold the stretch for longer periods of time. This is a common stretch technique in Yin and Restorative yoga classes. An example of this would be a standing forward fold with your arms and hands relaxed. The weight of gravity and the position of the body puts a natural stretch on your back, hamstrings and calves. This stretch technique uses the muscle spindle relaxation response.

3. **Active stretching:** This stretch technique is similar to passive stretching but we use the body to help us pull ourselves into the stretch instead of just relying on gravity. An example of this is Seated Forward Fold with our hands on our feet. Once you have a grip on your feet, you can use your arms to pull your torso forward increasing the intensity of the stretch on the hamstrings and lower back. This stretch technique can use reciprocal inhibition as well.

4. **Facilitated stretching**: Another term for this stretch technique is Proprioceptive Neuromuscular Facilitation or PNF. This technique briefly contracts the muscle being stretched then releases it and uses reciprocal inhibition to move into a deeper stretch. This technique is one of the most dramatic and is probably the fastest way to increase a muscle's flexibility by activating the golgi tendon organ. While it is the most effective it should be used sparingly to avoid putting too much stress on the tendons. Ray Long suggests using this technique once every three to four days on any one muscle group. Here are the steps for PNF:

    a. Stretch the muscle to its set length.

    b. Slightly contract the muscle you want to stretch about 20% of your maximum effort. Hold that contraction for 8-10 seconds.

    c. Relax the muscle for one breath.

    d. Use reciprocal inhibition to contract the opposite muscle and take up the slack created in the muscle to stretch deeper.

What's happening? When you contract the muscle that has already been stretched it puts more tension on the tendon connecting that muscle to the bone. This triggers the golgi tendon organ, which sends a message to the brain saying, "give me more slack in the muscle so we don't do damage to the tendon." Once this happens we engage reciprocal inhibition to enhance the relaxation response and use either our own body or someone else's to move us deeper into the stretch.

How much flexibility do I really need?
This is a common question among yogis. We see pictures of rubber backs and ballerina splits and think, "I need to be more flexible to do yoga well." The fact is that is not true. The more flexible a joint becomes the less stable it becomes. This is why I always teach naturally flexible students how to create strength and stability. So how flexible do you need to be? That depends on your lifestyle. For many people simply being able to touch their toes, fully extend their arms and move their spine with ease is good enough. How many times do you think during your typical day you are going to need to touch your toes to the back of your head? Probably zero! Your desired level of flexibility will most likely far exceed your needed level of flexibility, which is ok, but always work to create

balance in your body. As your flexibility increases, continue to build stability in and around your joints as well by seeking a balance between flexibility and strength.

Nervous System

The body's nervous system can be divided into two segments: the somatic or peripheral nervous system, and the autonomic or central nervous system. Arguably there is a third, the enteric nervous system, which relates to digestion, but for this context we will stick with the most common two. The central nervous system can then be further divided into its sympathetic and parasympathetic parts.

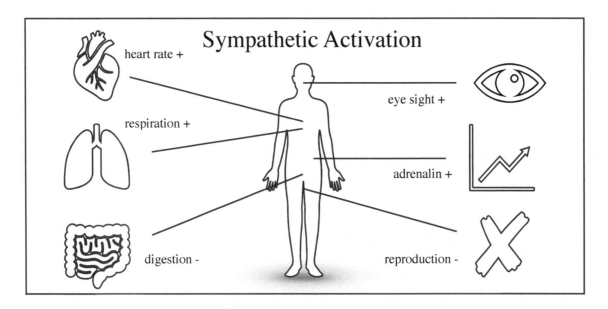

The peripheral nervous system is composed of a series of nerves radiating out from the spinal cord to the skeletal muscles, ligaments and tendons. It is largely responsible for conscious movement, (walking, throwing a ball, even taking a conscious deep breath). The central nervous system is a series of nerves radiating from the spinal column to different organs and glands in the body. Its functioning is done, for the most part, without our conscious control (regulating body temperature, monitoring heart rate, regulating hormones, etc.). The autonomic or central nervous system carries out its functions based on activation or suppression of either the parasympathetic or sympathetic system.

The sympathetic nervous system is sometimes referred to as the fight-or-flight response. In times of high stress this system is dominant. A series of physiological responses begin to take place to help prepare the body for a fight or to run from danger. Evolutionarily this has been a very important system for survival. During times of high stress the hypothalamus and pituitary gland, signal the adrenals to produce a series of hormones including epinephrine and cortisol. Cortisol is a stress hormone and epinephrine is adrenalin. These hormones, along with others, increase heart rate and respiration, dilate the pupils, shunt blood from the core to the limbs and hinder or shut down the digestive and reproductive systems. In situations of short-term stresses these physiological effects have proven to be highly effective for survival. However, they are not meant to serve as a sustained solution. If chronic, their health effects are devastating. Symptoms can be sporadic and unrelated and can include: depression, insomnia, short temper, energy loss, impaired digestion assimilation and elimination, decreased sex drive, impaired immune function, irritable bowel syndrome and more.

Parasympathetic dominance is referred to as the rest-digest response. It works on the opposite cycle of the sympathetic. Using a technique like breathing to create a more parasympathetic condition for the respiratory and cardiovascular system has a waterfall effect on the other systems in the body. This means that if you're consciously experiencing a sympathetic dominant state, simply pausing and taking a few slow deep breaths can shift the entire body two a more parasympathetic dominant state. While a parasympathetic dominance may sound more desirable of the two, if out of balance it too can cause health issues very similar to those of a sympathetic dominant state. The ideal is balance. The sympathetic system should be activated from time to time. This happens with many forms of exercise or mental problem solving, but these bursts should be relatively short and followed by more prolonged periods of parasympathetic/sympathetic harmony.

Your Body's Natural Anti-Depressant
In 2007 Chris C. Streeter and her team at Harvard Medical School released a study that showed the regular practice of yoga for at least fifty-five minutes a few times a week increased the level of the chemical GABA in the brain 27% and in some cases up to

80%.[33] GABA slows the firing of neurons making them less excitable and is known for reducing symptoms of anxiety and depression in the brain. Breath centered asana develops a sense of grounding, yielding to support, acceptance of what is, and awareness to where one really is in any moment. In my opinion the breath is the primary tool for everything you do on your mat. It provides focus in mind and body and a feeling of integration. Additionally, holding postures with breath can stimulate the release of GABA.

How you think about stress changes stress

In today's society, mental stress is probably one of our greatest sources of chronic stress. Stresses of the past used to be much more physical, fighting for our survival in a harsh and demanding world. We have now in many ways conquered the demands of the environment. The modernized world has eliminated many of the stressors of the past but there are new enemies in its place. The yoga philosophy outlines six emotional disturbances. These are: lust, anger, pride, greed, hatred and obsession. Their opposites then being: sexual restraint, happiness, humility, giving, love and non-attachment. Practicing these opposites begins to free us from the chains of the mind. One of the things I love about yoga philosophy is the principle that we must learn to become a master of our senses, not a slave to them. We do this by cultivating awareness to our current state and then slowly changing it to a more desirable one. There is no question this takes considerable time and thus quite a bit of dedication. The good news is the changes can start to be felt almost immediately.

Research now shows that simply changing the way we think about stress in our minds changes the body's physiological response to it. One of the responses your body has to stress is an elevated release of cortisol. While this hormone is necessary to cope with short-term stress physically, prolonged elevated levels of cortisol are associated with such things as impaired immune function and depression. When a stress has been alleviated, your body has stress recovery hormones. Two of these hormones are DHEA and nerve growth factor, both of which increase neuroplasticity which physiologically allows your brain to learn and grow from a stressful situation. The scientific term for this

---

[33] (Broad, 2012)

is stress inoculation. Higher levels of DHEA are connected to the reduced risk of anxiety, depression and more. The key is to have higher DHEA levels and lower cortisol levels. This elevated DHEA ratio to cortisol is called the growth index of your stress response.[34]

What's profound about this understanding is that a person's perception of how stress affects them influences their growth index. Those who view stress as making them stronger have a higher growth index. Those who see stress as "killing" them have a lower growth index.[35] Stress is the body's natural response to a challenging situation. If instead of viewing stress as crippling, a person views it as their body preparing to rise to the occasion, mobilizing energy and resources within them to perform at their best, their growth index improves.

We can change our brain chemistry with our thoughts and feelings. Meditation is a highly effective tool for bringing greater awareness to our current thoughts and beliefs. With practice the individual meditator is empowered to consciously shift their thinking and literally change their brain chemistry through the now widely accepted concept of neuroplasticity. Meditation uses primarily the senses of breath and awareness for focusing the mind. The goal of yoga is stillness, which is one of the primary healing drivers. The benefits of a regular meditation practice include: reduced stress, controlled anxiety, emotional health, enhanced self-awareness, improved attention span, improved memory, cultivates kindness, helps fight addiction, improves sleep, helps control pain, and can decrease blood pressure.[36] Simple gratitude and mindfulness based meditation have been shown to be quite powerful. Mindfulness is about accepting what is, starting where you are right at this moment and being ok with it. As Thich Nhat Hanh said, "If there is no mud there is no lotus." Meaning, we need to accept all of life's situations, even when they are difficult or challenging.

The breath is one of the most powerful tools that an individual has in order to bring about shifts in their physical and psychological state. Although respiration is typically regulated by the brain stem and under autonomic control, it can easily become a

---

[34] (McGonigal, 2015)

[35] (Department of Psychology, Yale University, 2013)

[36] (Mathew Thorp, 2017)

somatic activity. Increased respiration is one of the effects of a sympathetic state. By changing ones breathing pattern you can shift from a sympathetic to parasympathetic dominance. This would result in, lower heart rate, improved digestion, and a calming of the adrenal glands. Slow abdominal breathing also helps to tone the vagus nerves, and improve lymphatic functioning. When proper breathing techniques are combined with both asana and meditation practices, the benefits become even greater.

The Vagus Nerves

The vagus nerves are one of the 24 pairs of cranial nerves that extend from the brain down through the neck and throughout the torso. The vagus nerves are the main peripheral pathway for the parasympathetic nervous system and are important in controlling heart rate, blood pressure, metabolism, detoxification, cell repair, inflammation, digestive peristalsis, and other functions.[37] Vagus nerves have recently been discovered to have a role in affecting heart rate variability. According to research a resilient heart pumps at a slightly irregular rate. Having some variability in one's heartrate is a sign of a good balance between parasympathetic and sympathetic nervous system activation. Heart rate variability is the measure of the change in the heart's rhythm over time based on changes between sympathetic and parasympathetic activation.

Slow diaphragmatic breathing at a rate of 4-7 breaths per minute allows respiratory and cardiac systems to be more resilient to physical or psychological stress, improving autonomic balance.

Because vagus nerves innervate different organs and tissues throughout the torso it can be stimulated mechanically through movement. Yoga postures, especially chest opening postures like backbends, can improve vagal tone, parasympathetic activity and heart rate variability. Below is a list of activities that help stimulate the vagus nerve.

- Diaphragmatic breathing
- Smiling
- Heart Stretch
- Cat-Cow
- Compassion meditation

---

[37] (Shorter, 2014)

- Yoga Nidra / supine mindfulness meditation
- Diving reflex (ice or cold water on the face or hot/cold shower switch)
- Humming

Overview

- The vagus nerve has an inhibitory influence upon the sympathetic nervous system activity, creating a calming effect on the body.

- The vagus nerve extends from the brainstem down into your stomach and intestines, innervating your heart and lungs, and connecting your throat and facial muscles.

- Vagal tone is measured in the changes in heart rate that occur with the breath (Heart Rate Variability). Healthy vagal tone involves a slight increase in heart rate on the inhalation and a decrease of heart rate on the exhalation.

- Nerve fibers existing throughout your stomach and intestines are referred to as your enteric nervous system. This same system is sometimes called your "second brain." That is because 90% of those nerve fibers connect back up to the brain through the vagus nerve.

Proprioception and Sensorimotor integration

Proprioception is defined as the cumulative sensory input to the central nervous system from all mechanoreceptors (muscle spindles, golgi tendon organ, and joint receptors) that sense position and limb movements.[38] Mechanoreceptors feed the nervous system with information and are vital for the body to understand its environment in order to work out the most efficient movement. The ability of the nervous system to gather and interpret sensory information and to select and execute the proper motor response is called sensorimotor integration. What does this mean for our yogasana practice? Well, if the information is bad then the response will be bad, so if you are practicing a pose incorrectly the nervous system will build improper movement patterns. Once a movement pattern is established it is considerably harder to change than it was to create.

---

[38] (Michael A. Clark, 2008)

Motor Learning

Once you know about sensorimotor integration, the importance of learning the best movement patterns and alignment for postures as soon as possible is obvious. The body uses two different mechanisms to decide if a movement pattern is correct or needs to be adjusted.

The first is **internal feedback**. Internal feedback comes from sensors within the body. Proprioceptors act as a guide to establish proper force, speed, and amplitude of movement.

The second is **external feedback**. External feedback is information provided by some external source, such as a yoga teacher, or mirror. External feedback can provide you with either knowledge of performance or knowledge of results. Knowledge of performance is feedback provided during a yoga pose. This would be a hands-on adjustment or cue offered while practicing. Knowledge of results is feedback given after the activity has been completed. This could come as praise like, "Great Warrior II" or "that was excellent alignment."

It is a teacher's job to observe their class participants and offer both of these kinds of feedback to help solidify correct movement patterns in asana.

Consideration During Pregnancy

Whenever we get to this section of our teacher training I can instantly feel some of the students' nervousness. It's completely understandable. Many of them had never even thought about teaching an expecting mom and don't know what to do. I always reassure them that it's ok and they will be plenty equipped to handle it when it happens. The first thing I do is ask the women in the group, "If you were to learn that you were pregnant and you wanted to keep your yoga practice going through your pregnancy, what would you do?" Some of the common answers I get are: I would get online and start researching, go to the library or purchase books about yoga and pregnancy, and ask my doctor what to do. My reason for highlighting this is many of the pregnant women who come to a yoga studio for class have done one or all of these things. They have spent possibly hours researching the do's and don'ts of yoga and pregnancy, and possibly know more than you do about the subject by the time they walk in the door.

That being said, there are some key points to understand and consider if you yourself become pregnant and wish to continue with your practice, or are becoming a teacher and will lead future moms in class.

First Trimester: In the first trimester the baby is attaching to the uterus. This is the time when most miscarriages occur. A very gentle practice and pose selection is recommended. Some woman experience nausea, dizziness, and fatigue during this time period and don't want to practice. However, others feel well so if they are up to it, yoga is fine. As a teacher, you probably won't even know if a woman is pregnant during a majority or all of her first trimester. Many people wait for a few months before making the announcement and it is not physically obvious that a woman is pregnant during this time. I haven't come across anyone who wanted to take a chance and congratulate a woman on her maybe pregnancy because she was starting to look pregnant.

Second Trimester: This is the time when mothers usually feel their best. Energy levels are generally higher than the first trimester. Women can do anything they are comfortable with as long as they can breathe comfortably and deeply. At around five months you want to avoid lying on the belly or deep twisting. These movements become uncomfortable with a growing fetus occupying more and more space. They can also be potentially harmful to the baby. At this same time, mothers should avoid lying on their backs as well, as it can put pressure on the vena cava, which restricts the blood flow from the mother to baby. An easy answer to this is to use a single yoga block and a bolster to gently prop an expecting mother during any supine postures.

Third Trimester: Inversions should probably be avoided at this point due to lack of muscle tone in the back and belly. Deep backbends and twists should also be avoided. The hormone relaxin increases the water content in the collagen fibers of connective tissue making them more flexible in preparation for birth. Relaxin however, is not local to the pelvic girdle, it effects all of the joints. For this reason during the third trimester a mom should be more careful with pose selection and intensity so as not to injure an already destabilized joint. Some props will most likely be necessary to make poses more comfortable. Forward folds should be done with legs apart so there is room for the baby. It is suggested that once again the practice become gentler. Some pranayama, meditation, and mantra recitation can be very helpful in preparing for the birthing process.

It is important to highlight that if you are a yoga teacher. you are not a doctor. You should never give a practitioner medical advice. If asked a medical question you should refer them to their primary care provider.

Below is a list of warning signs to stop practicing and be sure to contact your doctor.

- Leaking of amniotic fluid
- Strong, regular contractions
- Nausea, vomiting, cramping
- Extreme dizziness or fainting
- Absence of fetal movement
- Difficulty walking
- Heart palpitations or rapid heart beat
- Uterine bleeding

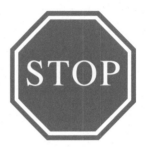

How to Breathe in Your Yoga Practice

Many new students ask "How am I supposed to be breathing during my practice?" With the breath being such an important part of yoga, this is a great question. The simple answer is, it depends. Not much of an answer at first, I know, but when we dive a little deeper, you will understand why this is true.

Our bodies breathe differently depending on our activities. If you were asked to run wind sprints up and down a football field, you would quickly notice that your breathing pattern increases dramatically. The term "sucking wind" expresses this exaggerated and fast-paced breath. In contrast, the breathing pattern of your yoga practice is encouraged to be slow and deliberate.

During a yoga class, we move through a sequence of pose categories. Generally speaking, it looks something like this: warm-up, standing poses, balancing (arm balances), backbends, forward folds, cool-down and Corpse Pose. A Vinyasa class follows an arc structure going from less intense to more intense and back to less intense. Our breath needs to be adjusted to accommodate this.

Pranayama is the fourth limb of Patanjali's eight-limb system of yoga. It precedes the yamas: ethical guidelines for how we interact with our environment; the niyamas, personal restraints; and asana, the practice of the poses of yoga. The Sanskrit word prana means energy, or the energy that is infinitely everywhere. Ayama means to stretch or extend. If we put the parts together, pranayama techniques work to stretch or extend the energy within us and even consciously move it in particular areas and directions. To this end, Pranayama uses breathing techniques sometimes accompanied by specific hand positions. Pranayama can also at times incorporate bandhas – energetic locks – in the body to concentrate the energy in specific areas. In this section, we will explore the science, philosophy and art of pranayama as well as look at the application of bandhas in both a pranayama practice and in our asana practice.

The Science of Breath

In order to better understand pranayama, and the way it affects the body, we need a basic understanding of the anatomy of the systems required for breathing as well as the physiology of how these parts relate to one and other (specifically the cardiovascular system and the respiratory system).

Breathing is essential: we can live for three weeks without food, three days without water, but brain damage can occur after only three minutes without oxygen. When we breathe, we are taking oxygen and other gasses into our lungs and transferring that oxygen to the bloodstream. It is then pumped by the heart throughout the body to aid in the process of metabolism: turning our food into energy.

Respiratory Anatomy

When we think of breathing, we primarily think of the lungs. However, the respiratory system is also comprised of bones, muscles, organs, and organ structures that all work together to allow us to breathe. When we take a breath in, the air is passed through the conduction passageways. Conduction passageways allow air to be purified, humidified and warmed or cooled to match body temperature. On exiting these passageways, air

Anatomy of Respiration	
Bones	Sternum Ribs Vertebrae
Muscles (inspiration/ breathing in)	Diaphragm External intercostals Scalens Sternocleidomastoid Pectoralis minor
Muscles (expiration / breathing out)	Internal intercostals Abdominals

then moves to the alveoli and alveolar sacs where it is moved in and out of the bloodstream through a process called diffusion.

The lungs are located inside the ribcage in what is called the pleural cavity. This sealed cavity allows the lungs to remain partially inflated at all times.

When we inhale, the primary breathing muscles of the external intercostals, and pectoralis minor muscles, as well as the secondary breathing muscles of the scalene and sternocleidomastoid muscles, work to lift and expand the ribcage. At the same time, the diaphragm contracts down towards the abdomen. These movements together draws air into the lungs.

When we exhale, the opposite movement occurs. The internal intercostals and abdominal muscles pull the ribcage down and in, and the diaphragm lifts up, forcing air out of the lungs.

Physiology of Breathing

The whole point of breathing is to bring oxygen from the outside environment to the cells and then carbon dioxide from the cells back to the outside environment. The volume that we breathe in and out is measured in different ways.

First is lung volume. There are four types of lung volumes. *Tidal volume* is the amount of air that moves in and out in one breath. This amount is variable depending on if we're exercising or at rest. *Inspiratory reserve volume* is the amount of extra air you can breathe in after a normal tidal inhale. *Excretory reserve volume* is the amount of extra air you could breathe out after a normal tidal exhale. Finally, *residual volume* is the volume of air that remains in the lungs after you've exhaled as much as you can.

Second is lung capacity. There are four types of lung capacities. *Vital capacity* measures the total amount of air you can breathe in and out. *Total lung capacity* is the sum of the vital capacity and the residual volume. *Inspiratory capacity* is the total amount of air you can inhale in a normal breath. Lastly, *functional residual capacity* is the sum of the residual volume and the expiratory reserve volume.

Parts of the Respiratory Passageways	
Conduction	Nasal Cavity
	Oral Cavity
	Pharynx
	Larynx
	Trachea
	*Right and left
*Within the lungs	pulmonary bronchi
	*Bronchioles
Respiratory	*Alveoli
	*Alveolar sacs

The final measurement is the anatomical dead space. This measurement is all the space between the mouth and the lungs which are filled with air but will never reach the bloodstream, because it never reaches the alveoli of the lungs. It includes the nasal passages, pharynx, larynx, trachea, right and left primary bronchi, and the branches of the bronchial tree that lead to the alveoli.

Minute Ventilation

Minute ventilation is the amount of air that is breathed in and out of the lungs in one minute. According to research, on average, this is 500 ml per breath x 12 breaths per minute = 6,000 ml per minute (about 1.5 gallons). This measurement, however, does not equal the amount of air that enters the bloodstream. If we account for the anatomical dead space, we could subtract roughly 150 ml per breath which at the end of one minute would leave us with an alveolar ventilation of 4,200 ml per minute. This is the amount of oxygen that actually enters the bloodstream. This is an important distinction to make because regardless of the breath speed or depth the alveolar ventilation will remain relatively the same. We can take faster, shallower breaths or deeper, slower breaths. While this varies the amount of breaths per minute, and the amount of air coming in per breath, the amount of air that enters the bloodstream actually remains the same.[39]

Nasal Laterality

Each of us has erectile tissue located in the nasal passages which swells at 60-90 minute intervals on either side of the nose. The result of this is we breathe more dominantly through the side that is not swollen at that time. This physiological occurrence is called nasal laterality. Furthermore, there have been studies that showed that when breathing dominantly through the left nostril, the right hemisphere of the brain is more active, and vice versa.[40] The right hemisphere of the brain is associated with nonlinear artistic and creative thought while the left hemisphere is associated with linear, mathematical and logical thought.

Interestingly nasal laterality also seems to have an effect on our nervous system with dominant right nostril breathing connecting with our sympathetic nervous system and left nostril breathing with our parasympathetic system.

Pranayama practices like Nadi Sodhana (alternate nostril breathing) were performed to bring balance to the energies flowing through the main left and right energy channels that weave up the spine. These channels are associated with masculine and

---

[39] (Coulter, 2001)

[40] (Robin, *A Handbook for Yogasana Teachers*, 2009)

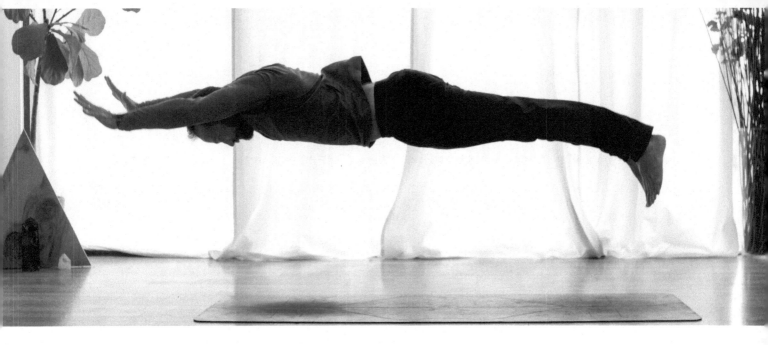

feminine energy which correlate directly to the qualities of the left and right hemispheres of the brain.

Cardiovascular Anatomy

The cardiovascular system is composed of the heart and blood vessels. The heart, as we know, pumps blood through the body. The heart is composed of the atria which collect blood coming into from the veins and arteries. The right atrium takes in deoxygenated blood returning from the body, while the left atrium collects oxygenated blood coming from the lungs. The ventricles, which are larger than the atria, pump blood out of the heart. The right ventricle pumps deoxygenated blood to the lungs, while the left ventricle pumps oxygenated blood to the body[41].

The average person's heart rate at rest is between 70-80 bpm (beats per minute).

Blood vessels are a closed circuit of tubes that move blood to and from the heart. Blood vessels are divided into two different categories.

Vessels that transport blood to the heart are called *veins*, while vessels that transport blood away from the heart are called *arteries*. Larger arteries become smaller the further they get from the heart and divide into arterioles which then branch out into microscopic capillaries. It is in the capillaries that oxygen is transported to the cells and waste products removed.

Venules collect waste products and distribute them back to the veins where they are eventually cleaned and moved back to the heart.

---

[41] (National Academy of Sports Medicine, 2008)

The *cardiorespiratory system* is the combination of both the cardiovascular and respiratory systems together. Without these two systems working, the body could not turn chemical energy – food) into mechanical energy – work).

The human cell is the basic building block for life. There are approximately 100 trillion cells in the human body working at all times to carry out their particular function within the larger system. It is within the mitochondria of the cell that energy is produced. Properly oxygenating the blood is essential to the efficient functioning of each cell. Without oxygen, cells cannot carry out their metabolic function, meaning they cannot produce energy. If cells become dysfunctional or die the entire body and all of its systems are effected.

Breath effect on The Body

The process of breathing is also intimately connected with the rest of the kinetic chain: the skeletal, muscular and nervous system. A normal relaxed breathing pattern is observed as the belly expanding on in inhale and contracting on an exhale. If we experience regular high levels of stress, our breathing pattern will change. In a stressful state, the breath becomes faster paced and can lead to an inverse breathing pattern where the chest expands more on an inhale and the belly contracts. An inverse breathing pattern over-activates the use of secondary respiratory muscles and under activates the primary ones. If dysfunctional breathing persists, it can create inadequate joint motion in the spine and rib cage, cause headaches, dizziness, neck pain, back pain, feelings of anxiety, and altered carbon dioxide and oxygen blood levels. A regular yogasana and pranayama practice helps to correct dysfunctional breathing or prevent it all together.

Beyond Yoga

Nutrition and Lifestyle

The Upanishads divided food into 16 different categories: Ten parts were classified as wastage, five parts affected the energy of the mind and one part is vital for the intelligence. Food can have a positive or negative effect depending on surroundings, geographical and climate conditions, and a person's constitution.

The yoga approach towards nutrition is best known through its sister science of Ayurveda. In the Ayurvedic system there are three main constitutions or doshas. Each dosha has specific characteristics which describe a person's overall physical appearance as well as address things like temperament and the way they digest food.

Foods are classified into three different categories: sattva, raja and tamas. Sattva represents the balanced and meditative aspect; rajas represents the energy to accomplish and create; tamas represents inertia and decay.

Sattvic foods: are fruits and vegetables

Rajasic foods: onions, garlic, and pungent spices

Tamasic foods: alcohol, meat and junk food

From the viewpoint of yoga, the five organs of perception: eyes, ears, nose, tongue and skin are the gateways to the mind. In order to better control the mind, we need to properly nourish the organs of perception. This means the ears should be exposed to soothing music, the eyes to soft natural light or peaceful scenery. The nose should be exposed to fresh air and nutritious and delicately flavored foods. The skin should be kept clean, soft and supple.[42]

The below guidelines are based off of my own research on the subject of holistic nutrition. They are not diet specific but rather general guidelines to help you navigate decisions surrounding food and cooking.

1. Eat whole foods that have been humanely and/or organically raised.

2. Store foods and water in glass containers avoiding brass, tin and aluminum.

3. Cook using stainless steel, cast iron or ceramic.

4. When using oils be sure to use the appropriate oils at the appropriate temperatures.

5. Avoid the consumption of soy.

6. Avoid the consumption of sports drinks, sodas, and other sweetened and caffeinated beverages. Instead consume fresh juice, water and herbal teas.

7. Drink half your body weight in pounds, in ounces of water daily (120lbs = 60oz. of water)

8. Limit your consumption of processed white flour, milk, sugar and salt.

------

[42] (Iyengar B. , 2008)

9. Learn more about your dosha type and/or Metabolic Type™ when choosing your foods and their ratios.

The year is 1901. It's 6am and the sun is just coming up over the horizon. A man rises from his bed, gets dressed and heads downstairs. There, he eats a warm meal, freshly prepared with whole foods. When done he steps outside and takes a deep breath of the crisp morning air. There are animals to be fed, trenches to be dug and repairs to be made. He will spend the day pushing, pulling, bending, squatting, lunging and twisting throughout all of the activities of his work. Before the day is done, he will have two more fresh cooked meals and find himself sitting with a good book beside the flicker of a lamp light. By 10pm, he will be in bed getting a good night's rest in preparation for the next day.

In my book, *Good Being Good Living*, I use the acronym FARMERS to stand for: Food, Air, Rest, Movement, Environment, Resources, and Stressors. Each of these seven categories contributes to our health and together they make up a holistic approach to good living.

In the past six years, I've had the opportunity to coach a wide range of people, from yogis to some of the military's most elite warriors. Through it all, there is one very important theme I've learned. If you want a practice to be sustained, keep it simple. Below are a few of the key points, summarized from the book.

Food: Eat More of Less

Eat more of the foods with fewer ingredients. Another way to say this is to eat more whole foods. There are only six different food categories: meat, vegetables, fruits, nuts, seeds and dairy. You will find that most of these items are found around the perimeter of the grocery store, so that's where you should shop. Spend less time in the aisles and more time on the perimeter.

Air: Take a Deep Breath

Of all seven categories, this is probably the most important. Our breath has a profound impact on our nervous system and our nervous system affects everything from our stress level to our ability to digest our food. Take time throughout the day for a deep breath. Two or three deep breaths can swing your body from a "fight or flight" state to a "rest-digest" state. This will improve mental clarity, digestion, sleep, energy levels and more. Here's what you do. Go to a local office supply store and purchase some brightly colored, little round circle stickers. The kind you would use for labeling the price of something at a tag sale. Stick them in multiple locations around your house or work, on the periphery of your usual lines of sight. Every time you catch a glimpse of one throughout your day, pause and take a deep breath.

Rest: Recharge the Battery

There are three types of rest: active, passive and total. An example of active rest is a gentle yogasana class; passive rest is listening to some relaxing music or reading a book; total rest is sleeping. Balance your day with forms of active, passive and total rest. Many of these activities have other health benefits as well. When it comes to sleep, try to wake with the sun and turn off bright lights by sundown. For thousands of years, our sleep/wake cycles have evolved in close connection with nature. It wasn't until the very recent invention of the light bulb that we have removed ourselves from Mother Nature's light and consequently removed ourselves from the natural rhythms of our bodies. Getting enough sleep gives the body time for physical and mental repair, which is essential for good health.

Movement: Fix the Kinks, and Functional First

Our body was built to move. With proper movement the joints are stronger, the heart and lungs more efficient, hormones, digestion, energy, and mood are all improved. That being said, in order to enjoy these benefits and avoid injury, you should properly align the body first. One of the great things about a regular yoga practice is that if it is sequenced well, the stretching and strengthening effects of the postures can help bring musculoskeletal deviations back to balance. If you are experiencing pain it might be best to work with a trainer, corrective exercise specialist, physical therapist or symmetry practitioner one-on-one to correct the deviations. Once the body is properly aligned think about functional movement. Functional movement is: pushing, pulling, bending, squatting, twisting and lunging. Using your own body weight or free weights are great places to start. Avoid the use of exercise machines that isolate specific muscle groups and allow the rest of the body to relax. This is not how your body moves through space so should not be how the average person trains.

Environment: You Live in Three Worlds

There are three major worlds we operate in: our work world, our home world, and our recreational world. Each one of these worlds carries with it its own characteristics and responsibilities. Your work world is a place that you earn a living, but should also be a place that is healthy for your mind, body, and spirit. Your home world is a place to rest, nourish and connect with family and friends. It should be safe, clean and comfortable for you to live in. Your recreational world is a place to have fun, exercise, connect socially and relax. This world is the easiest one to engage in practices that do not support your health. Take stock of your three worlds and begin to make adjustments so they become environments where you can feel supported and grow as a human being.

Resources: Time and Money

What are the two things we don't ever have enough of? Time and money. It is important to your health that you are honest and clear with yourself on how much of these two resources you need to be happy and where they should be invested. If you look at the first five categories, it doesn't cost you a dime to breathe differently and it doesn't take much time either. This is why I say it's the most important. It has the greatest effect with the least impact on your resources. While it always feels like we don't have enough time, the real issue is when we aren't suing our time to do the things we want. Getting into the regular practice of setting clear and meaningful intentions will change the way you see time and how you use it.

Stressors: Stress is Good

All people experience physical, physiological, psychological, emotional, intellectual and spiritual stress. The key is to convert negative stress into positive stress. There are innumerable conditions associated with or directly caused by too much stress on the body/mind.

Everything is stressful and that's a good thing. Right now, you are in a field of gravity that is pulling your body towards the earth. This is a physical stress. If you ate anything today, your body is working to digest it. This is a chemical stress. If you're processing the information in this book, you're experiencing a mental stress. Everything is stressful. But it's important to keep our stress in proper balance and to view it as making us stronger.

Life is dynamic; you are an expression of life, so you too are dynamic, an intricate symphony of systems all striving towards perfect harmony with one and other. Like an orchestra, if one instrument is out of tune the entire ensemble is affected. Eating a healthy diet, properly exercising, breathing exercises and rest all contribute to balancing stress in the body and alleviating some of its negative effects.[43]

Losing Weight with Yoga: The Myths and Truths

Currently about 33% of the US population is considered to be obese (having a BMI score greater than 30). It is no surprise then, that there are numerous yoga programs out there marketed as being able to help you lose weight. But is yoga an effective practice for weight loss? In order to answer this question appropriately a number of factors need to be taken into consideration.

---

[43] The sections covering the FARMERS model were extracted from my previous book, *Good Being, Good Living*, Lulu Publishing, 2014

First there are many different styles of yoga. Some focus very little on physical postures of asana while others do. How these different disciplines might help with weight loss needs to be considered.

Second we have to determine how weight loss is achieved. If weight loss were merely achieved by intense exercise then the answer to our question would most likely be no. In a study done at Duke University, Hatha Yoga practitioners were compared to a similar group that participated in aerobic exercise on a stationary bike. At the end of the study those who used the bike saw an increase in their VO2 max[44] of 12%. The Hatha yoga participants showed no increase at all.[45] Another study done in 2007 concluded that Hatha Yoga represents a low level of physical activity, similar to walking on a treadmill, and was not significant in improving or maintaining health or cardiovascular fitness. The one exception was that sun salutation postures do contribute some portion of sufficiently intense physical activity and showed some improvement in cardio-respiratory fitness in unfit or sedentary individuals.[46]

But given that weight loss is achieved not just by intense exercise but also includes other factors like nutrition, stress and lifestyle, then the answer could be yes: yoga can help with weight loss. Anyone who has practiced yoga regularly for an extended period of time knows that it has the power to "work on you" in ways you aren't always aware. When I first started yoga I was 225 lbs., using chewing tobacco, and drinking more then I should. Today I am 185 lbs., haven't touched tobacco for a long time, and no longer drink alcohol. I didn't start practicing yoga with the intention of all this happening, it was just part of the process.

Yoga has been shown to improve mindful eating, increase intuitive eating and spirituality, improve health behaviors, improve mood and self-compassion, and promote healthy lifestyle behaviors even when they are not prescribed.[47] Additional research

---

[44] VO2 max (volume of oxygen uptake) is a measurement of how efficiently your heart and lungs work together to create energy.

[45] (Broad W. J., 2012)

[46] (Marshall Hagins, 2007)

[47] (Tosca D. Braun M. C., 2016)

shows that yoga is a valuable tool for helping people improve their dietary and exercise behaviors over a long period of time.[48]

The practice of yoga postures is not the best choice for improving ones cardiovascular fitness when compared to other activities like swimming, cycling, and running. However the benefits towards helping to achieve long term weight loss goals is absolutely evident, and yoga is a powerful tool for anyone looking to improve their overall health.

Yoga, the Mind and Post Traumatic Stress

The American Psychological Association defines resiliency as "the process of adapting well in the face of adversity, trauma, tragedy, threats, and even significant sources of stress – such as family and relationship problems, serious health problems, or workplace and financial stresses."[49] By this definition if an individual is not able to "adapt well" then they are then they are vulnerable to suffering when faced with all the difficulties that life inevitably throws up. The tools and techniques of yoga, breathing practices, and meditation balance stress in the body and use its positive aspects to make us more resilient. Furthermore, they are surprisingly easy to integrate into daily living with profound results.

The human brain is a fascinatingly complex organ that has been evolving for millions of years. Today the number of possible combinations of your 100 billion neurons firing or not is approximately 10 to the millionth power. As a point of comparison, the estimated number of atoms in the universe is only 10 to the eightieth.[50]

Through the process of evolution humans developed three distinct survival strategies. The first was creating defined boundaries between themselves and the world. The second was to maintain stability in order to keep physical and mental systems in balance. The third was approaching opportunities and avoiding threats in order to gain things that promote offspring and avoid death or injury.[51]

---

[48] (Tosca D. Braun B. C., 2012)

[49] (Charney, 2018)

[50] (Rick Hanson PH.D. with Richard Mendius, 2009)

[51] (Rick Hanson PH.D. with Richard Mendius, 2009)

As a necessary faculty for survival, we have what scientists call a negativity bias. What this means is we are biologically hard wired to look at and remember the negative events more easily then the positive ones. When a negative event is experienced it is flagged by the hippocampus and stored for future reference. As Richard Hanson puts it, "your brain is like Velcro for negative experiences and Teflon for positive ones." This is because through the course of evolution, the negative events had the most drastic impact on survival.

When you see something that is potentially dangerous your brain sends a signal to your amygdala which in essence is like an alarm bell that starts the cascade of nervous system and hormonal reactions in the body. Simultaneously, what you see is sent to your pre-frontal cortex for more sophisticated analysis in order to ascertain whether or not it is an actual threat. However, that process works much slower than that of the amygdala so our nervous system is triggered before our conscious mind can reason if the correct response.

While the evolution of the brain and nervous system have certainly proven to be beneficial for survival, the overall health implications of chronic stress can be dramatic. Post-Traumatic Stress effects an estimated forty-four million Americans with the numbers for US combat veterans being even higher. It is estimated that one in three military combat personal, roughly 300,000, individuals experience PTSD.[52]

Unhealthy but common ways of coping with these symptoms include alcohol and drug dependence and reckless behavior. On the other hand, realistic optimism, facing fears, social support, altruism, religion and spirituality, finding role models, proper exercise, meditation, cognitive and emotional flexibility, and connecting an individual with purpose are all healthy, effective practices to becoming more resilient .[53] It just so happens that these practices are not only good for building resiliency towards PTSD but also for those who suffer from TBIs (Traumatic Brain Injuries), and almost all these tools are taught in yoga, too.

---

[52] (Richard C. Miller, 2015)

[53] (Charney, 2018)

Using Yoga to Build Resiliency

The yoga practice has existed for thousands of years. It is now widely understood that one of the basic principles of the practice is to help calm mind and body. More recently, research has shown that yoga practices, including meditation, relaxation, and physical postures, can reduce autonomic sympathetic activation, muscle tension, and blood pressure, improve neuroendocrine and hormonal activity, decrease physical symptoms and emotional distress, and increase quality of life.[54]

The value of yoga for individuals coping with trauma is to be able to increasingly self-regulate with yoga tools and practices, and to develop mindful resilience in the face of traumatic reminders, and life's challenges. Yoga can provide a safe, predictable and controllable experience for this to take place.

Traditional yoga and Ayurveda models help us to see practitioners as individual points of light, within the entire context of their struggle. It's important to see and feel the whole person, on physical, psycho-emotional and spiritual planes, whose internal world (subtle body) effects and is affected by family, society and more. This idea is basic to yoga: to help a practitioner discriminate between their true, deepest self and the trauma that is caught in the memory of the five levels of human experience: physical, energetic, mental, intellectual, and divine.

---

[54] (David Emerson, 2009)

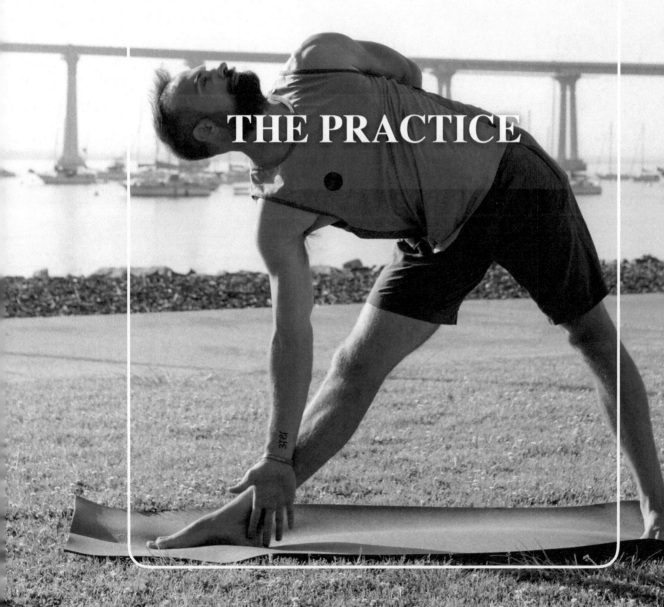

THE PRACTICE

THE PRACTICE

Asana

Yoga has a beautiful way of always meeting us where we are. It simply and elegantly outlines a set of practices carefully refined over thousands of years.

Asana Comes from the root ās, meaning to sit. It is a description for how we should take our seat to prepare for meditation. That seat is one that is steady and comfortable (sutra 2.46). While this definition still holds true, the word asana has become better known in the West as meaning the many different physical postures of yoga.

Foundational Qualities of Yogasana

The practice of postures has evolved throughout the years. The Hatha discipline of yoga had a strong emphasis on purifying the body in order to achieve spiritual liberation, and part of that practice introduced some yoga poses. In the early 1900s when Krishnamacharya opened his yoga school in Mysore, India, he taught a wide range of poses and created the term Vinyasa. Vinyasa means to move consciously from the roots, *Vi* – "in a special way" *nyāsa* – "to place."[55]

Krishnamacharya taught that the asana practice has three essential qualities: Breath, Body, and Mind. These three qualities are woven together into one flow, like smaller streams merging into a greater river. He continued to support Patanjali's earlier description of asana as needing to be balanced between two qualities: sthira (steady and alert) and sukha (to remain comfortable).

Yogasana so powerfully connects to daily living that, in my opinion, the lessons it has to teach are innumerable. Today there are thousands of poses with new ones being created all the time. The physical practice of asana has been a well-studied topic since becoming more popular in the West. Research has gone on to show many of the benefits as well as the potential side effects (contraindications) to traditional practices. Some of the benefits include improved flexibility, improved sleep quality, improved digestion, greater confidence and self-image, reduced stress levels, improvements in circulation,

---

[55] (Desikachar, The Heart of Yoga, Developing A Personal Practice, 1999)

116

improved joint health, improved mood and decreased anxiety. Some of the benefits can also be contraindications if practiced improperly. For instance, inappropriately stretching the body, moving the joints in a position that could damage connective tissues, inappropriate sequencing, and poor teaching techniques.

When you build a house, one of the first things you need to do is secure the foundation. If the foundation is strong, it will support the house for years. If it is weak, it will crack, and everything on top of it will become weak and more likely to fall. The same could be said for your asana practice. If the foundation for your practice is weak, then you are more prone to struggle in your postures, to give up or even to become injured. Another interesting thing to note about a foundation is that once the house is built over it, it is rarely noticed. The foundational principles presented here are not flashy. They can be integrated into the practice of both a beginner and a more advanced yogi.

In my years of teaching and studying yoga, I've found the following three principles to be essential for building a strong foundation. Each principle has two parts. The first relates to the gross body. This is the anatomy of form. The second refers to the subtle body. This is the anatomy of the mind, energy system, and spiritual body. I will explore both aspects of each principle in detail. The three principles are as follows:

1. Maintain strength in your core
2. Lead with your heart
3. Never collapse into a pose

Principle 1: Maintain Strength In your Core
The body's core musculature is comprised of four layers, each one building on the one below it. From the deepest moving outwards, they are: transverse abdominals, internal oblique, external oblique and rectus abdominals. The abdominals are crucial to maintaining proper posture, supporting the torso and connecting the passenger unit (torso and upper extremities) to the motor unit (hips and lower extremities). These muscles are also the primary muscles for breathing. The transverse abdominal acts like an Olympic weight belt around the lower back, where many back injuries occur. The transverse abdominal connects to the vertebrae of the lower back and wraps around the waist to the navel, ribs, and hip bones. This deepest layer of abdominal musculature is probably the

most important when discussing our asana practice. The engagement of this muscle has two critical functions. One, it stabilizes the lumbar spine by preventing over flexing or extending. Two, it creates a lock, or bandha, through the torso that can help move energy through the body or isolate other joints in an asana. Let's look at each of these in more detail within the context of standing postures.

The engagement of the transverse abdominals stabilizes the lumbar spine limiting the possibility of over flexing or extending. This is best seen in standing postures such as Warrior I, Warrior II or Crescent Warrior. Let's look at Crescent. When in Crescent Warrior, the front knee is bent to 90 degrees so that your thigh is parallel to the ground. The back leg is extended with the heel of the foot lifted. The torso is lifted, and the arms are extended up overhead. In this position, the hip flexor on the back-extended leg is stretched.

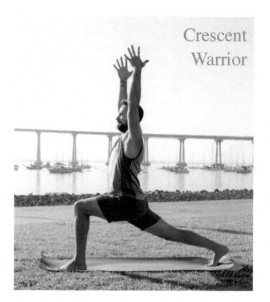

Crescent Warrior

This action pulls the pelvic bones into an anterior or forward tilt. With excessive anterior tilt in the hips, there is compression of the vertebrae in the lower back. To alleviate this compression, you need to engage the transverse core. This engagement tilts the hips back slightly, relieving any excessive pressure in the lower back. The same motion occurs in Warrior One.

The spine is designed to work on all three planes of motion: Sagital [flexion/ extension], coronal [abduction/adduction], and transverse [internal and external rotation]. It is comprised of a series of vertebrae that stack one on top of the other and are divided into five sections. The top of the spine from the skull to roughly the top of the shoulders is called the cervical spine. The cervical spine is comprised of seven vertebrae labeled C1-C7. The cervical spine connects to the thoracic spine which is a series of twelve vertebrae labeled T1-T12. The thoracic spine connects to the lumbar spine. It is a series of five vertebrae labeled L1-L5. From the hips to the bottom of the pelvic floor is the sacrum. This is a series of five fused vertebrae terminating at the final section the coccyx.

The spine has an "S" shape to it, which is entirely formed by the late teenage years. The S shape allows for a wider range of motion through flexion and extension. The curves of the spine are identified as lordotic or kyphotic. A lordosis or lordotic curve when looking from the side looks like a backward "C." A kyphosis or kyphotic curve is the reverse. The cervical spine is lordotic, the thoracic spine is kyphotic the lumbar spine is lordotic again, and the sacrum and coccyx are kyphotic.

When we move into a backbend, the curve naturally begins in areas of lordosis. The spine is already in position to take this motion, and the sections of the lumbar and cervical spines have the widest degree of movement in this direction. The problem with this is we can extend this lordosis too far and compromise its stability. This can create issues with intervertebral disks and the nerves radiating out from the spine. The disks are like little pillows between the vertebrae that provide a cushion for comfortable movement. If the disks are disrupted or ruptured, it creates severe pain.

OK, enough about spinal anatomy. What does any of this have to do with your practice?

During a backbend, you will naturally want to move from your cervical and lumbar spine to achieve the "depth" or at least the "feeling" of depth in the pose. This is fine since the body has been designed to move in this way. In the average person, the lumbar spine has a 35° range of extension, the cervical spine a 75° range of extension, while the thoracic spine only has a 5° range of extension[56]. However, without proper counteraction, injury can occur.

When practicing Camel Pose (Ustrasana) for example, if you relax the abdominals during the backbend, you will surrender the weight of your upper body onto only a few disks in your lumbar spine. Your lumbar spine already supports roughly 80% of your body weight. Your hips will tilt forward, lifting the top of the sacrum. The thoracic spine, which is not designed to have a wide range of extension (5° on the average person), will reach its max and lock. The locking of the thoracic spine will draw all forces into the lumbar spine, compressing the back and possibly causing injury.

---

[56] (Robin, 2009)

However, if you counter the forward tilting of the hips by drawing the navel up and in, engaging the core, you will keep the sacrum from lifting too far, and you will also stabilize the thoracic spine through a secondary engagement of the diaphragm. Doing this will allow you to find a broader and more supported range of motion in both the lumbar and thoracic spine because they will not be compressed, but lifted, creating more space to move.

This principle shows up in asana after asana: standing postures, backbends, balancing postures, twists, and more. Without engaging the core, you are putting yourself at a greater risk of injury and you won't have balance of strength (sthira) and ease (sukha) required for proper asana expression.

When you draw the navel up and in towards the diaphragm, you create Uddiyana bandha, also known as Gate Lock. Bandhas are used in yoga to move or retain prana in a certain area of the body. Prana is the life force that flows through all things (explained in greater detail later). By engaging certain bandhas one can intensify the fire (agni) within in order to clear blockages in the energy body. It's important to note that this particular bandha has no functional application to our asana practice, as it is activated through the retention of your exhale. However, it is incorrectly used as a common cue by yoga teachers to get students to engage their core muscles. You should always be breathing when performing asana, so this bandha is reserved for your pranayama practice. For that reason I use the cue "modified Uddiyana bandha" when I teach and then take the opportunity to explain the difference to any student who is interested.

The word core has a double meaning. In any yoga practice, you want to explore and maintain the integrity not just in your physical core, but also your core values, virtues, and ethical guidelines. Two of the eight limbs in Patanjali's Yoga Sutras are the yamas and niyamas. The yamas are ethical guidelines that govern your actions in the way you relate to others. The niyamas are ethical guidelines that govern how you treat yourself. Each of these is then broken into five subsections. I have simplified them below, but the essence of their meaning remains intact.

Yamas:

1. Ahimsa: Non-harming

2. Satya: Truthfulness

3. Asteya: Not taking what is not yours

4. Brahmacharya: Sexual restraint and responsibility

5. Aparigraha: Non-attachment

Niyamas:

1. Sauca: Cleanliness both inside and out

2. Santosha: Acceptance of the way things are

3. Tapas: Self-discipline and willpower

4. Svadhyaya: Self-inquiry and study of wisdom literature

5. Ishvarapranidhana: Selfless action and surrender to God

The regular practice of the yamas and niyamas builds an unshakable "core" of values.

Principle 2:

Lead with your heart

When I instruct my students to lead with their heart, I am not using the anatomical location of the heart, which is found on the left side of the chest. Instead, I am referencing the energetic location of the heart or heart chakra, located at the center of the chest.

It seems to be the more natural tendency for students to lead with their heads. After all, most of the senses are found consolidated in this sphere upon your shoulders. Your organs for sight, smell, hearing, and taste are all right there in your head. However, yoga teaches you not to be a slave to your senses but instead to be the master of them. Instead of leading with your head, and thus in many ways your senses, try to lead with your heart. Doing so helps to draw the senses inward (pratayahara), one of the key practices to achieving liberation (moksha). Regardless of the body's position in space, it is best, in my opinion, to lead with the heart.

Let's look at a few examples. In plank position, the heart is in line with the shoulders, hips, knees, and ankles. People with a weak core will have a tendency when transitioning from plank to low-plank, as in a Chaturanga Dandhasana, to drop their hips, putting pressure on the lower back. Repeating this movement over and over can lead to injury because of the compression it adds to the intervertebral discs of your lumbar spine.

However, if you lead with the heart and keep the hips lifted and in line with the shoulders, you maintain integrity in the core (principle 1) and the lower back is protected.

When transitioning from low plank to an Upward Facing Dog, the same two principles apply. The core needs to be engaged to protect the lower back, and the heart instead of the head should be the focus of your lift in Up Dog. The heart lifts and pulls forward as the hands pull back, creating length in the spine. The tendency to lead with the head, lifting the gaze up and back, can restrict blood flow to the basilar artery, discussed in more detail later.

In forward folding postures like Paschimottanasana, Uttanasana, Janu Sirsasana and more, lifting the heart center creates length in the spine; and the core draws in, keeping you from collapsing into your lower back. These movements allow you to forward fold safely and increase the stretch in the desired area.

In twisting postures, the heart becomes the center axis that you twist the body around. Imagine the heart center as a ball which the torso rotates around in numerous directions. Again, by leading from the heart center in a twist, you don't collapse into your twist (principle 3). Instead, when you draw your navel up and in (principle 1), you stabilize the spine and create more space in the thoracic vertebrae to twist more deeply, but also with more stability. If you lead with the head, you put more of the twist into the cervical spine and do minimal twisting through the rest of the back.

All asana should maintain a delicate balance between strength and ease. Standing and balancing postures require a lot of strength in the lower body, so you must seek to find more ease in the upper body. The concept of strength and ease will be covered in more detail is principle three.

You never hear anyone say, "That person has a lot of head!" Instead, the expression is, "That person has a lot of heart!" What does this mean concerning yoga? Yoga teaches you to think and move from your heart. Yoga asks you to understand that all living things desire to be loved, including you. When you "have a lot of heart," you understand this, and you understand that we are all the same. The higher your pedestal, the more treacherous the fall. The more treacherous the fall, the more fear you have of falling. Fear is the great enemy of the heart. Operating from the ground, equal to all others, is the only place you can be free. From here, on the ground, we can ascend together, and the only place to go is up, together as one. A true yogi understands that consciousness will vary from person to person and time to time. You must step down to the lowest level you find and extend a hand to lift up. In yoga philosophy, the term Kivalya is used to describe one who exists in this way. A mastered yogi, one who has achieved sustained enlightenment, or in Buddhist terms Nirvana, consciously chooses to walk the world, in it, but not of it. They remain in the world to help others.

To extend a hand and as the Buddha said, "remove the arrow of suffering from one's heart", we do not need to be self-righteous, but loving. A true yogi knows this must be done within oneself first. Identify your enemy as it lives and breathes inside of you. Only then do you have the ability to fight for another.

The heart chakra is one of seven chakras commonly studied in yoga philosophy. It is the 4th chakra, below the throat, third eye and crown chakras and above the sternum, navel, and root chakras. It sits in the middle and is represented by a triangle pointed up, and overlapped by a triangle pointing down. Each chakra has related categories of influence over the physical and mental bodies:

Physical issues: Shallow breathing, high blood pressure, heart disease, cancer, asthma, bronchial pneumonia, upper back pain, shoulder pain, breast issues.

Mental/emotional issues: Fears of betrayal, co-dependency, hatred, bitterness, grief, anger, jealousy, fear of loneliness, inability to forgive.

Yogasana helps us open the energy centers associated with the different chakras. Many of the poses work with specific energy centers to help open the channels of energy, allowing the prana to flow more freely. In the Kundalini practice, practitioners perform specific asanas to experience the Kundalini energy rise up the spine from the root to the crown chakra. By practicing asana with a special focus on leading with the heart, you energetically amplify your ability to work through some of these blocks, both physically and emotionally.

Principle 3:

Never Collapse Into a Pose

Correct asana as taught by such yoga masters as TKV Desikachar and BKS Iyengar is a delicate balance between strength (sthira) and ease (sukha). I have mentioned the balance between strength and ease within asana practice several times. It's key! The body must maintain a level of strength and effort to consciously place itself into the position. However, that effort must be countered with an equal level of ease. If it is not balanced, the body becomes fatigued, and the mind becomes uneasy. Desikachar suggests that a good way to assess if you're maintaining this balance is to always to be aware of your breath. In a balanced state, the breath flows evenly and comfortably. The breath as he says in *The Heart of Yoga*, "is your teacher." If you can maintain a comfortable ujjayi breath (common pranayama breathing technique), then your mind can remain free to explore the deeper lessons the asana has to offer.

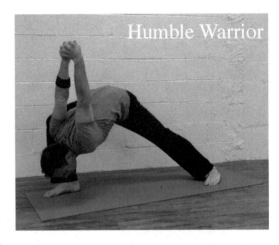

Humble Warrior

This directly relates to the third principle: never collapse into an asana. When you collapse into an asana, you lose the balance between the strength and ease.

Take, for example, Humble Warrior. In this asana, the legs are in a Warrior One position, and the torso is folded forward with the shoulders inside the front knee. If you were to collapse into this posture, you would lose the integrity in the core. There would be increased stress placed on the piriformis and other hip rotators, and the rounding of the spine would compress the diaphragm, impeding a smooth and even flow of breath. A similar posture is the common Runners Lunge.

In this pose, the front foot is placed at the top of the mat with both hands resting inside of it. The back leg is extended straight. The posture is designed to help open the hips. Some people like to explore a deeper stretch in the hips by coming down onto their forearms. If this pose is practiced with all three principles, the stretch is felt in the intended location, the hip. If we collapse, we would again see a rounding of the spine, taking the movement into the vertebrae and out of the hip socket, thus eliminating the intended stretch. The back leg when relaxed will tend to externally rotate, dropping the pelvis off to one side, placing more weight on the upper extremities to that side, and eliminating the balance from the left and right sides of the body.

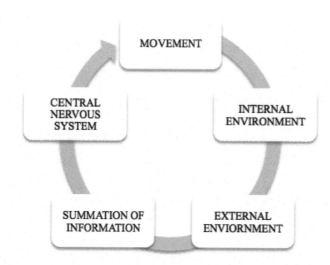

In Upward Facing Dog, if you collapse into the pose, the head sinks down between the shoulders. The hands will externally rotate placing pressure on the carpal tunnel; the core will remain loose allowing the hips to touch the ground and compress the lower back. The legs can also internally rotate with the heals falling out. This positioning of the legs may not be a danger in and of itself, but when you combine it with the upper body, the transition from here to Downward Facing Dog makes the body much more susceptible to injury.

In a balancing posture like Warrior III, if we collapse, of course, the obvious thing that happens is we fall out of the pose. The less obvious is a rounding of the spine, a drop in the head, and a drop in the extended leg hip. These collapses all move us further and further from the ideal position of the asana and make the body much more susceptible to discomfort and possible injury to the deep six hip rotator muscles. The coordination of movement is the responsibility of three main systems of the body: the skeletal system, the muscular system, and the nervous system. These three systems together are called the kinetic chain.

The nervous system is constantly receiving external and internal information from both the surrounding environment and other systems within the body. It relays that information back to the central nervous system, spinal cord, and brain, which in turn responds with the appropriate corresponding signal to activate specific muscles in order to initiate movement. This movement of muscles, of course, also moves the bones. The brain works quite hard during movement, especially new and more complex movements for which it has never built a program.

In all of its wonder, the brain has an amazing ability to conserve energy. When we repeat a movement over and over the brain builds a program for that movement. Think about when you brush your teeth or wash your body in the shower. You almost always perform the movements in the same way. By creating these programs, the brain is freed to think about other things. It's like placing the body on autopilot. While this is a great tool for physical evolution, it can be a roadblock to your yoga practice. One of the great benefits of your asana practice is building awareness.

When you collapse into an asana, you move less consciously. When the body is at total rest, there is much less energy required for coordinating movement or maintaining posture, and thus there is more space for the mind to wander. A wandering mind lacks focus, and focus is key to your progression along the yogic path, both on and off your mat. An unfocused mind is an undisciplined mind, and this is the cause of much of our suffering as human beings. The constant flood of thoughts we experience every day has more influence over our moods than we often realize.

If you were to reflect upon your thoughts throughout the day, you would notice that many of them fall into two categories: reflecting upon the past and imagining events of the future - rehashing and rehearsing. This type of thinking is a unique gift we have as human beings. Rehashing in and of itself it is not necessarily harmful, unless it leads to judging yourself or others. Rehearsing in and of itself is not bad, unless it leads to stress and anxiety about what is to come. The problem is, often times our rehashing and rehearsing does lead us into emotional states that challenge our happiness. As the Buddha said, "the disciplined mind is trained like an archer. Each thought is focused on its bull's eye." The mastered yogi lives in "the power of now" – also the title of Eckhart Tolle's most famous book. When the fluctuations of the mind are stilled, the observed and observer dissolve. The separation of the "I" self merges with the divine in all things and frees us from suffering. After all, yoga evolved as a discipline of the mind. While only one limb of the Yoga Sutras is asana, there are three dedicated to working with and controlling the mind (Pratayahara, Dharana, and Dhyana).

A clear and focused mind, attentive to the bodies position in asana, knows when it is not properly balanced between strength and ease. This knowledge allows a student to make a conscious alteration to the pose. With this principle it is be the ability to engage more fully in a posture so as not to collapse into that pose.

The 3 Principles Working Together

These three principles—integrity in your core, lead with your heart and never collapse—like the limbs of Patanjali's Yoga Sutras, are best practiced together, and in fact, are intimately connected. The integrity of the core stabilizes the back, allowing lift and length of the spine as well as movement from the hips, where it should be happening. When you practice this way, you can more easily lead with your heart, instead of your head. If you are leading with your heart, then it becomes almost impossible to collapse into poses. The practice of yoga requires what Gandhi referred to as "the patience of a man [woman] trying to empty the sea with a teacup." Persistence is key to your progression. Every step forward is a step towards new understanding, and every pause is an opportunity to reflect. With your Vinyasa, your steps become more conscious. The choices you make are of your own will. Yoga is accessible to everyone. Desikachar tells us, "The world exists to set you free." Approach your practice with the words of these great teachers in mind and heart. Apply the three principles each time you step onto your mat, and you will have a foundation strong enough to support you for years.

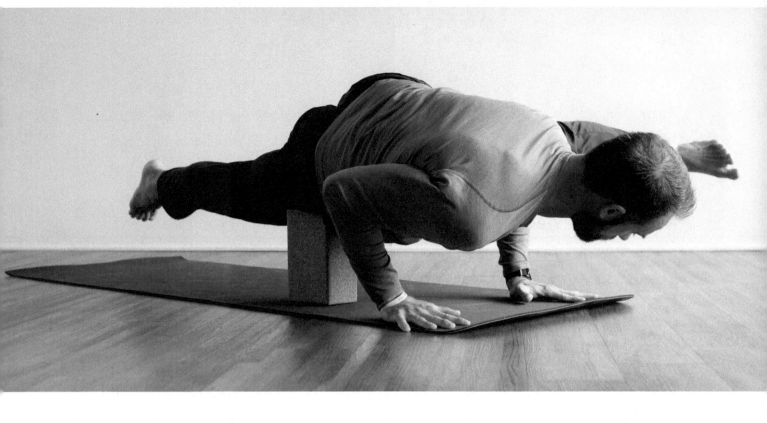

Using Props in Your Practice

Almost all studios have them, tucked away on a shelf or in a closet somewhere. When you're new to yoga, you don't have any idea what they are. Blankets, bolsters, straps, blocks, wedges, rolls, balls, etc. Yoga props are common in most studios, but how often are they used? New practitioners certainly don't grab them on their own, because they wouldn't know what to do with them. What about as a teacher? Do you use these asana aids in your classes? The correct application of yoga props is a great addition to a class as a tool to help improve a practitioner's experience. Let's review some of the more common props, their function, benefits and practical applications.

BLOCKS

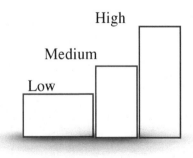

Blocks come in a couple of different sizes. They range in material from softer foam to more firm cork or wood. They are a highly versatile tool as an asana aid. Blocks can be adjusted to varying heights depending on the side placed on the ground or the number of blocks used. Blocks can also be used to stabilize certain areas of the body.

Function: *Brings the ground up or extends a limb or body part down to the point of support. Stabilizes an area of the body by connecting it to the ground, through the block.*

Benefits: When we stretch the body to its limits, we can find ourselves holding unnecessary tension that restricts our ability to find a deeper expression of a pose. Having a block to place or rest a part of the body on relieves this tension which creates space to consciously choose, with greater ease, how to work with the muscles to balance the energy in the pose.

- Downward Facing Dog: Blocks under the hands provides space for lengthening through the back of the legs and opening the chest.

- Upward Facing Dog: Blocks under the hands allows for a broadening of the chest and opening of the front plane of the body.

- Balancing poses: Blocks under the hands in balancing poses like Warrior III, and Balancing Half Moon, brings the ground up allowing for greater length through the torso, providing an ideal position to breathe smoothly and completely in the pose. When working with Tree Pose or Eagle Pose, a block can bring the ground up and serve as a place to rest the toes of the lifted leg to help stabilize the balance.

- Revolved poses: When twisting, practitioners can sometimes go too far. When this happens, there is a shortening of the breath and the body. Think of a washcloth. If you keep twisting one end in one direction and the other end in the opposite direction, it slowly starts to shorten until it's a tight ball. Using blocks under the bottom hand in twisting postures gives some support and lift, which lengthens the torso and takes some strain off of the legs allowing for greater ease and openness through both the upper and lower body.

- Supine poses: Resting on top of blocks can help to open the front plane of the body in a more restorative way. Placing a block at the back of the heart for Supported Fish pose, or under the sacrum in Supported Bridge are both examples of this (the number of blocks used and height can be varied depending on ability and desire). Placing blocks under the knees in Reclining Cobbler's pose can alleviate pain in the hip sockets and allow for a deeper release of the adductor (groin) musculature. Blocks under the feet in Bridge pose create a deeper inversion. Blocks under the knees in Supine Twists set the stage for us to take a practitioner into a deeper twist with an adjustment, without pushing them too far. Blocks on the belly help to teach abdominal breathing, serving as a point of reference to fix the mind and train the muscles of the core.

STRAPS

Straps come in different lengths, materials and have different clasps. Deciding on the intended use of the strap will help you determine the length needed.

<u>Function:</u> *Straps serve to connect two points, often bringing limbs together. They can also be used to support the body.*

<u>Benefits:</u> Sometimes the level of flexibility a person has limits them from achieving the full expression of an asana. A strap can help with this, allowing the practitioner to feel the benefits of the pose. Bringing limbs together like hands to feet or hands to hands in binds can help a practitioner work to increase their range of flexibility and joint motion.

<u>Practical Applications:</u>
- Bringing limbs together: When trying to bring the hands together behind the back as in Cowface Pose, Bound Extended Side Angle, Birds of Paradise or a Bound Crescent Twist, limited shoulder flexibility may limit a practitioner's ability to achieve hand-to-hand contact. By holding on to a strap, they can find a grip that their body currently allows and slowly work the hands closer together providing a comfortable stretch to the shoulder joint. In Dancers pose a strap is turned into a loop and can loop around the lifted foot and held in the same side hand to pull deeper into the quadriceps of the lifted leg. In King Pigeon, a strap can be used as a loop as well. Looping the strap around the lifted ankle and held with the same side hand or both hands to help pull the lifted leg in towards the head. In Seated Forward Fold a strap can be used to wrap around the feet and held with the hands to ease the torso forward and down while

keeping a flat back (this same technique can be applied to other Seated Extended Leg poses as well).

- Supporting the body: In Boat pose a strap can be turned into a loop wrapping around the lower back and the arches of the feet. By pressing into your feet, you keep the natural curve in your lumbar spine allowing the chest to lift and open. In Reclining Cobbler's pose, you can wrap the strap around the feet and lower back in a loop to help achieve the same result in the low back and surrender deeper into the hips. In Legs Up the Wall pose a strap can be used around the upper legs to allow for a release of muscular energy in the legs creating a more restorative expression.

BLANKETS

Blankets can be folded and rolled to different sizes and shapes making them a highly versatile prop. They come in a variety of colors as well. The most popular are usually the "Traditional Mexican Yoga Blanket," measuring at 74"x52." They are softer than blocks and can be folded to a lower height to serve a similar function.

Function: *Blankets are used to provide support often when seated or underneath a part of the body that would otherwise be uncomfortable without it.*

Benefits: Sometimes the range of motion required to reach the full expression of a pose safely is not available to a practitioner. This can stress the joints and even cause pain. A blanket can be used to alleviate pressure off of a joint, providing more stability and comfort in the pose. Blankets are quite versatile in their ability to fit the contours of the body by being rolled and or folded into different shapes. They can also be used to cover the body in Savasana to keep it warm.

Practical Application
- Seated: Blankets can be used to sit on to bring the hips into better alignment. You want your knees to be level with your hips or lower. A blanket lifts the hips, taking pressure off of the hip socket providing a more comfortable seat.

- Forward folds: In seated forward folds a blanket under the sit bones allows for greater ease in establishing anterior (forward) tilt to the hips which helps to lengthen the spine and move deeper into the fold. Some practitioners experience discomfort under the ankles in Child's Pose. A blanket can be rolled and placed under the ankles for support.

- Kneeling: Blankets can be used under the knees as additional cushioning to provide more comfort in a pose like Camel.

- Savasana: Some practitioners experience discomfort in their lower back while lying supine due to an excessive anterior tilt of the hips that put pressure on the vertebrae of the lumbar spine. By rolling a blanket and placing it behind the knees, you create a posterior tilt to the hips and alleviate the pressure and pain to the back.

The examples given are of course not an exhaustive list but provide you with a basic understanding of a few of the more popular yoga props used in a classroom setting, their benefits, function, and examples of their practical application within specific poses or pose categories.

Some disciplines of yoga like Iyengar employ the use of props much more heavily, while other styles of Vinyasa do not. Experiment with props in your practice to build a deeper understanding of how they work for your practice.

How to Customize Your Practice with Four Principles

We all come to our mats from a unique place. David Keil, the author of *Functional Anatomy of Yoga*, refers to our current state based on past experience as converging histories. He explains them in this way. "Our converging histories make us exactly who we are at this moment. . . Every moment that we live we choose experiences, activities, and relationships that become part of our sea of converging histories. They become part of us." Keil outlines six major histories. They are human evolution history, genetic history, learned parental behavior history, activities history, injury history, and spiritual history. Each one of these has played a role in shaping you – literally, physically and spiritually – into the person you are right now.

It is virtually impossible for a yoga teacher in a group yoga class to know and understand each student's converging histories. For this reason, it is challenging to customize a practice to best serve each individual. Since this is the case, you can empower yourself to customize your own practice using these four principles.

1. Time: The amount of time you stay in certain postures increases the difficulty level. Take Chair Pose for example. The longer you hold the pose, the harder it becomes. Your legs start to burn, and your back begins to fatigue. You can adjust the time you hold the pose to decrease the intensity and struggle. There are some exceptions of course like some postures supported by props or supine poses that do not require much strength or flexibility.

2. Strength: The amount of strength required in a pose increases its difficulty. For example, a handstand is challenging to do if you do not have the proper shoulder, back, and core strength. Being inverted in this way challenges these muscle groups. Based on your converging histories you may want to find a modification or alternative pose.

3. Flexibility: The more flexibility a posture requires, the more challenging it can be. For example, full splits require a high level of flexibility. This makes this pose incredibly

difficult for many. For some, it feels like a resting pose. Props can be used to help support the body as one slowly opens their hamstrings, hips and psoas.

4. Points of Contact with the Ground: Generally speaking, the fewer points of contact with the ground the more challenging a pose can be. Take Crescent Warrior for example. If the back knee is on the ground in Modified Crescent, many people find the pose easier to balance. When in full Crescent, and the back knee is lifted it becomes more challenging. If you were to then step up into Warrior III, it would be even more challenging, as you are now standing on one foot. In contrast to this think about Savasana. High points of contact, little flexibility and little strength required. Ahh. . . That sounds nice.

When you understand these four principles, you can walk into any class at any level and modify the postures to best work for you and your converging histories. BKS Iyengar once said, "when I practice yoga, I do not practice the poses of yesterday or tomorrow, I practice the poses of today." The next time you're on your mat observe the

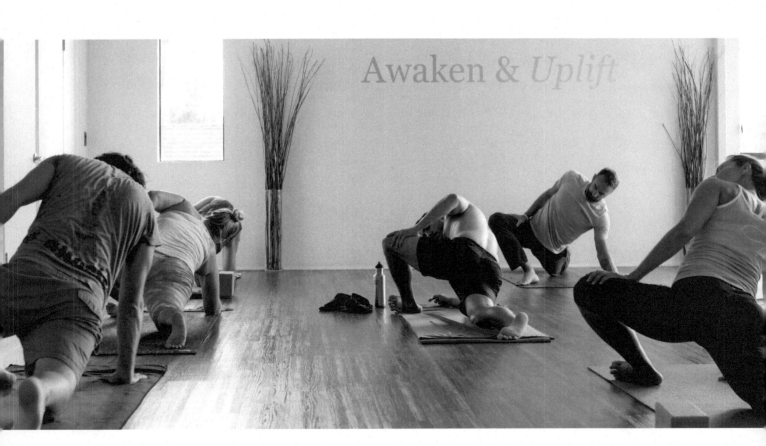

movements and think about how you can adjust the poses to fit your practice, not yesterday or tomorrow, but today.

More Difficult

INCREASE: Strength, Flexibility & Time
DECREASE: Points of Contact

Less Difficult

DECREASE: Strength, Flexibility & Time
INCREASE: Points of Contact

Taking Your Practice to the Next Level

Throughout my years of teaching, I've heard lots of people express an interest in "taking their practice to the next level." I would say that there are many ways to do this, but most people are referring to their ability to perform more complex and difficult yoga poses.

One way to improve our ability to do the postures of yoga is, of course. . . to do the postures of yoga. With a regular mat practice, we become stronger and more flexible over time. The more you practice the faster you will improve in strength, flexibility and overall ability.

That being said, there are lots of other ways for us to improve our strength. It has been my experience that exercising with resistance training, HIIT (high intensity interval training), and calisthenics exercises can speed up the strength building process and when done in balance with a regular asana practice show huge benefits. Because asana uses our body's own weight against the force of gravity as resistance, I like to practice a hybrid between traditional vinyasa and calisthenics exercises I call yogasthenics.

For examples of yogasthenics exercises and workout routines along with much more you can view and subscribe to my Youtube channel.

Another way that we can take our practice to the next level is through a regular meditation and pranayama practice. We've already discussed in detail the anatomy of pranayama and some common practices. Integrating these into your daily yoga practice or other daily routines will help you to understand both yourself and yoga with greater depth and wisdom.

The Five Things You're Doing That Cause Injury

The rapid growth of yoga as a physical practice in the West has captured the interest of inquiring scientific minds. The result has been a huge number of scientific studies exploring both the benefits and side effects yoga has on our bones, joints, muscles and minds.

Unfortunately, much of the research never makes it to those where it will have the most profound impact: the average yoga studio teacher and practitioner. I have listed below some commonly taught movements or cues that should be either avoided or adjusted.

1. Basilar Artery Constriction

In the back of your head, slightly above and in front of the brain stem, is an artery called the basilar artery. The basilar artery distributes blood throughout the brain. It is formed from the joining of the two vertebral arteries in combination with the Cerebral Arterial Circle. Research shows that cranking your head back in a position like Upward Facing Dog can constrict the flow of blood through the basilar artery. In the most extreme cases, this can cause a stroke. In less severe cases, symptoms can include, vision problems, vomiting, difficulty breathing, arm and leg weakness and sudden falls[57]. Any pose in which the head is put into an extreme position forward or backward could cause constriction of this artery and should be avoided. Some of the most common examples of this in yoga are Upward Facing Dog and Camel pose. I tell students who I see cranking their heads back in Upward Facing Dog to pick a spot where the wall at the front of the room meets the ceiling. When practicing Camel pose I encourage students to tuck their chin more towards their chest and keep their gaze on the ceiling instead of the wall behind them.

---

[57] (Broad, 2012)

2. Pulling Your Shoulder Blades Away from Your Ears

One of the primary reasons your shoulder has the range of motion that it does is because of the anatomy of the shoulder blade. In fact, if your shoulder blades were not able to rotate and elevate you would not be able to extend your arm much more than 90 degrees from your side. A very common cue in yogasana is to draw your shoulder blades away from your ears in Downward Facing Dog. Doing this works against your body's natural anatomy. When your arms are extended overhead the medial spines of the shoulder blades rotate down placing the glenoid process (the socket) of the shoulder blade under the head of the humerus (arm bone). This provides greater stability. Pulling the shoulder blades away from the ears moves the shoulder blades out of this position and puts more pressure on the soft tissues (ligaments, muscles and tendons). This position provides less stability and could cause injury to the soft tissues over time.

Instead, push the mat away with the hands, engaging your upper back. Press firmly through all ten finger tips and try to gently pull your mat apart, left to right. This will broaden your back and keep your shoulders in a safe and stable position.

3. Neck Rolls

The vertebrae of the neck are very close together in comparison to those of the lumbar and even thoracic spine. Each one is separated by a cartilaginous intervertebral disk. Transverse processes and facets link the vertebrae to one another as well as to the connective tissues that give the spinal cord its tensegrity.

A very common warm-up movement is neck rolls. While this type of movement may feel good for the musculature of the neck, it is not good for the spine itself. Both Coulter and Robin warn against such movement as it can rub the bones of the spine against one another, grinding them. While many people don't go close to their limit, this is still a very unnatural movement for the neck and can cause injury to those doing them for the first time. Coulter in his book, *Anatomy of Hatha Yoga*, highlights the unnatural movement of neck-rolling with this example:

"Let's say you are looking down into your lap and suddenly your attention is called to a bat in the upper right corner of the room. You don't have to think. Your head will move quickly and safely in a straight line to face the object of your concern, and muscles and restraining ligaments will protect you from going too far. By contrast, if you connect the two points with a fast neck roll instead of linear motion, you will immediately see why such movements serve to be treated with caution (Coulter, 2001)."

Instead of neck rolls, move the neck through a single plane of movement at a time. Right to left, side-to-side, up and down. It is always best to move slow and listen to your body.

4. High Hinge Folds

There are two different anatomical points of bending. One point of bending is from the lumbar and lower thoracic region, which creates a collapse of the chest and changes the relationship between the pelvis and lumbar spine. In a standing forward fold, the pelvis tips back (posterior) while the spine flexes forward. This puts unnecessary pressure on the intervertebral disks. Pre-existing disk injuries will be made worse and new injuries can be created when folding in this way. Movement from this area referred to as the upper hinge. There is insufficient activation of the psoas when bending from the upper hinge, and it leaves students prone to injury. [58]

The other, more desirable point of bending, is from the hips. This movement is one that encourages the yogi to lead with the chest, maintaining integrity in the core and maintains an ideal relationship between vertebrae of the lumbar spine and pelvis. This point of movement is referred to as the lower hinge. When bending from the hips the transverse abdominals (deep core muscles) activate and stabilize the vertebra of the lumbar spine. Keeping the spine in an elongated position when folding forward or backward protects the intervertebral disks from bulging or rupturing.

---

[58] (Robin, 2009)

During a yoga practice, we move often from standing to folding as in Uttanasana. Folding from the high hinge can be detrimental to anyone who has spinal spondylolisthesis (slipped vertebra), spinal stenosis or disk issues. Folding from the high hinge causes the back to round as you move from standing to forward fold or from a forward fold to standing. This compresses the disks and could exacerbate an existing disk issue. It is therefore preferable to keep the spine as neutral as possible and hinge from your hips. If your hamstrings are tight, you may need to bend your knees slightly to allow this to happen. Bending your knees will free your pelvis, allowing it to tilt forward which in turn will neutralize your lower back.

5. Square Knee Chair Twists

The sacroiliac joint or SI joint is the point where the hip bones meet the sacrum. This joint is held together by a number of ligaments. The sacrum can move into nutation (forward movement) and counternutation (backward movement). Because of its position at the base of the spine, movement of the sacrum is intentionally limited in order to make it more stable, which is what makes it able to support the weight of the upper body.

A common instruction in yoga class is to keep your knees in line with one and other when in a Chair Twist. Doing so stretches the ligaments of the SI joint that are trying to hold the sacrum and pelvis together. Doing this repeatedly can result in pain. The sacrum simply isn't designed to have flexibility in this area, and increasing flexibility here compromises its ability to be stable.

To avoid this, simply allow the knee on the opposite side from the direction you are twisting in to move forward slightly. This will allow the pelvis to move and keep the ligaments of the SI joint from being strained. You can apply this same principle to other twisted poses like Marichyasana I and III.[59]

---

[59] (Lasater, 2015)

Pranayama Practices

Ujjāyī: "What clears the throat and masters the chest area."
Technique: Take a comfortable seat with your lips gently closed. Press your tongue to the roof of your mouth, and just behind the upper teeth. Create a slight constriction in the back of your throat, as though you were about to whisper. Breathe in and out like this, ensuring your inhales and exhales are of equal length.

Ujjayi breathing is the most common type of pranayama used during a vinyasa practice. It helps to build heat in the body by swirling the air at the glottis before entering and exiting the body. Ujjayi breathing also engages the sense of touch, since we can feel the constriction in the throat, and the sense of sound, since we can hear the breathing. This type of breathing helps us to practice pratyahara, the fifth limb of yoga, which is the act of drawing the senses in from the outside world to the inner world.

Variations:

Anuloma Ujjāyī –Breathe in through the nose, then close one nostril and breathe out through the other. Alternate back and forth.

Viloma Ujjāyī – Three-part breath (wave breath) in through the nose and out through the nose while maintaining the constriction in your throat.

Nādī Śodhana: Nadi "Channel" Śodhana "Purification"
Technique: Take a comfortable seat. Place the thumb and ring finger on either side of the nose. Partially close the right nostril and breathe in. Then switch the fingers to block the left nostril and breathe out through the right nostril. Keep the left nostril blocked and breathe in through the right nostril. Reverse the pressure of the fingers and breathe out through the left nostril. Continue to repeat in this manner as long as you're comfortable. When you're ready to conclude your practice, release both nostrils and take a soft breath in and out.

Alternate nostril breathing is a technique for cleansing the two sub-nadis of Ida and Pingala (explained earlier). This breathing technique helps bring balance to the energies of the body – creating a more sattvic state of mind.

Kapālabhātī: Kapāla "skull" bhātī "That which brings lightness."
Technique: Take a comfortable seat. Take a deep breath in through the nose. Exhale, in short, diaphragmatic breaths, pulsing the breath out through the nose. Your breath should be short, rapid and vigorous. Continue for anywhere between 10 to 100 pulses.

Kapalabhati pranayama is sometimes difficult to get the hang of in the beginning. Each breath out is a short rapid exhale that continues for multiple pulses. With each pulse, there is a natural recoil of breath that comes back in. However, the recoil in is less than the pulse out, so eventually the lungs empty. With this pranayama technique, one inhale might have anywhere from 10-100 mini exhales. It's important to use the abdomen to press the air out, not the chest. To help keep track of your pulses you can place your hands on your knees in closed fists. Every ten pulses out you extend a finger. Once one hand is open you've reached 50 pulses; both hands open 100. This technique is one that helps loosen and release stuck energy.

How should I sit?

While some people say that you must be in a seated lotus position to achieve the greatest movement of energy, it is my opinion that not everyone can sit in lotus, and even if you can, you may not be able to sit there for long because it becomes uncomfortable. If this is the case, then our pranayama practice could be cut short as a result of discomfort. I think that the best position is one that is comfortable and stable. Some possible positions may include:

- ✓ Seated Lotus
- ✓ Sitting in a chair
- ✓ Seated cross-legged
- ✓ Kneeling (on or off heals)
- ✓ Lying Supine
- ✓ Sitting on a bolster, zafu or another similar prop

Even without practicing a formal pranayama, there are multiple techniques to focus our attention, stabilize the fluctuations of the mind, and balance the body's many systems (including energetic ones). Here are a few suggestions.

Flow: Focus your attention on the rhythm and flow of your breath as it moves in and out. Start to notice the nuances of your breathing and even out the inhales and exhales so they are of similar length.

Sound: Listen to the sound of the breath as it moves through the body. Using Ujjayi pranayama increases the noise of the breath so it's a good technique to use here. Earplugs are also a great tool to amplify the sound of the breath within, allowing you to focus on it with greater ease. If you don't have earplugs, you can simply try plugging your ears with your fingers.

Placement: Consciously visualize sending the breath to a particular area of the body, or while practicing, notice if the breath moves into a specific area on its own. You can visualize prana filling that area as you breathe.

Gaze: With your eyes closed, direct your inner gaze up and towards the middle of the brow, the area of the sixth chakra. Holding the gaze here helps to focus the mind. Another option is to hold an image in your mind's eye and try to keep focused on that image without distraction.

Mudra: The Sanskrit word mudra means "gesture" or "seal." In this context, we are referring to hasta-mudras or hand gestures that affect the subtle energy body.[60] Jnana mudra, "the seal of wisdom," is a simple hand mudra that calms the mind and reverses the outward flow of prana back in toward the body. To 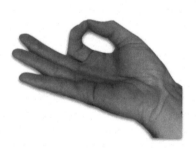 engage this mudra, rest your hands on either knee if seated, or beside you on the floor, if supine. Gently bring the tips of the thumb and index finger together to touch with the

---

[60] (Carroll, 2013)

palms facing up. If you begin to lose focus your fingers will separate. As soon as you notice the separation of the fingers, slowly bring them back together to touch.

Counting: Place the tip of your thumb in each section, of each finger, on each hand. With every breath move the thumb to the next section. A count of twelve is traditionally used. Once you reach twelve, you can either count back down to one or start over again at the beginning. Alternatively, if you have a mala, you can count the beads on the mala as you progress from one breath to the next.

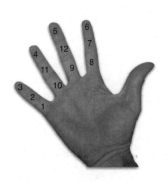

Bandhas

The word bandha is similar to mudra in its definition as a "seal." Other translations include "lock", "bind together" or "close". Bandhas are traditionally used to help intensify the fire (agni) within, burning up any energetic trash so it may be eliminated. The three major bandhas covered here are:

- Jalandhara bandha: Throat Lock
- Uddiyana bandha: Gate Lock
- Mula bandha: Root Lock

Jalandhara bandha is located in the cervical spine and back of the throat. To engage this lock, lift the crown of the head in order to lengthen the spine. Draw the head back and lower the chin towards the chest. You should still be able to breathe comfortably as the muscles at the back of the neck lengthen the cervical spine. This lock can be used during certain seated or standing postures as in Siddhasana or Janu Sirsasana.

Uddiyana bandha is created in the area where the thoracic and lumbar spine meet. To engage Uddiyana bandha, contract the abdominal muscles on an exhale, lifting the navel up and in. Contract the rectal and lower back muscles to help stabilize this lock.

This bandha is only engaged when the exhale is retained. A common miscue in asana is to use the term Uddiyana bandha to describe the action of pulling in the navel to engage the core and stabilize the back. While this engaged core position is often crucial for the safety of our practice, it is not a true Uddiyana bandha because we must continue to breathe throughout our yogasana practice.

Mula bandha is located in the lower abdomen, pelvic floor, and base of the spine. This bandha is engaged when we engage the perineum, pulling the musculature of the pelvic floor, up and in. A cue often used to help practitioners with this engagement is to imagine that you had to cut off the flow of urination. Mula bandha can be utilized throughout our yogasana practice in particular standing postures such as Chair Pose and Warrior I.

Bandhas can amplify the effects of the practice and improve the overall benefits but should be used with caution and do not need to be integrated into every pose or pranayama practice. Start slowly and incorporate them a little at a time, paying close attention to the way you feel physically, mentally, and energetically.

Pranayama is a vital part of the yoga practice and one that should not be overlooked. While here in the US, we are particularly focused on the asana, the most physical part of yoga, it is important to approach classical yoga from all eight limbs. Like the spokes on a wheel, if one spoke is weak the tire will not be able to maintain its shape, and the ride will be very bumpy.

BECOMING A TEACHER

BECOMING A TEACHER

Introduction

The practice of yoga has been studied for thousands of years. Its lineage of teachers is long, and many of them have left us with great wisdom to learn from as we step on the path beside them. This path requires the utmost dedication and commitment.

Becoming a good yoga teacher is demanding of your time and your energy. It will test your self-discipline while bestowing the rewards of living the life of a dedicated, soul-centered leader.

Teaching yoga is a gift that we earn through practice. Coupled with awareness of our actions and always learning, there is no replacement for experience.

That being said, there are plenty of things for you to learn before you even step onto your mat to lead others. I have outlined here what I believe to be the key components of teaching yoga. With time and practice, you will feel more and more confidence in what you're doing and how you're doing it. With enough practice, you will not just lead a class but be able to experience being part of the energy of the room as mind, body, and breath come together in greater harmony and flow.

Ground Rules

We are teachers, not masters. We hold a neutral space for our students to discover their own power and ability to self-heal. When we teach, we need to come from the truth of who and what we are as human beings. We need to discover our own voice without mimicking or copying others. We allow ourselves to become more vulnerable, thinning our ego boundaries and letting our spirits expand. We do this by practicing what we preach. If we can do this, we foster the ability to fully connect with other human beings. A connection is vital when teaching yoga.

Practitioners come to yoga for many reasons, including to heal and to grow. We as teachers are there to give of ourselves, but not to "save" or "heal" another human being. That mentality strips the practitioner of their own power. We need to be mindful and use a dialogue with our practitioner that promotes the message that we are guides, aiding them in their own development. We do not teach from atop a pedestal but from the mat beside them. Each student's journey is an intimate one. We are there to embody and set the example through our words, actions, and the energy that we emanate.

We need to start from a place of authenticity and honesty and go from there. When in doubt, just breathe with the class. Make sure to allow space for the student's to have their own experience. Be mindful not to have expectations of the class. The class will go where it goes, and that's ok. During class, make sure to focus on holding the energy of the room, especially when it drops, and be supportive.[61] Each student comes in with their own energy, their own beliefs, their own past, their own ideas and their own expectations. If you notice yourself becoming self-conscious, take your energy to your heart. Speak to alignment and foster the ability to align breath with movement. Bring awareness to what is in the head and heart. Pay attention to the dynamics of the class. Are they fighting? Are they making weird faces or grimaces? When this happens, speak to breath and be conscious of temperature, tempo, difficulty, and intensity. It may be the class itself, or it may be that the students are working through their own struggles. It is the job of the teacher to find the balance.

Lastly, take joy in teaching. Teaching Yoga is a celebration of being human, being alive, and sharing love and life with one another through movement.

Developing as an Authentic Principle-Based Yoga Instructor

We become authentic by developing our skill, power, self-awareness, and energy, with the courage to be introspective and honestly assess our morals, strengths and needed areas of development. We need to ask for and appreciate feedback from other teachers, practitioners, family, and friends. The frameworks we use to develop as a teacher incorporate the following:

Spiritual and Philosophy Base: This is a combination of scholarly study and integration from experience. Through study and experience, we use dialogue with our students that is simple, clear, and demystified. More importantly, we share this

---

[61] This is a skill that is learned over time. It is difficult to teach because it is a subtle awareness that is felt by a teacher.

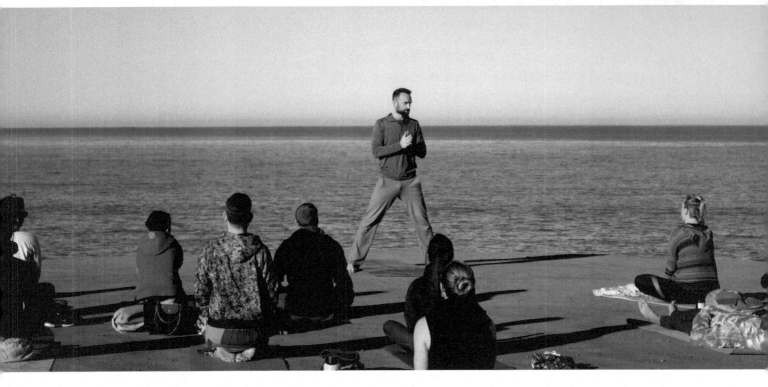

knowledge not from the head, but from our being, our wisdom and direct experience. This means that we focus on speaking from our hearts in class, rather than from our head. One way to do this is by placing your hand over your heart as you speak to the class. When you speak from the heart, the energy is literally felt and experienced by the practitioners. When we speak from the heart, separation is removed, teacher/student is removed, and a connection emerges.

Knowledge of the Science of Asana: This is the study of alignment, biomechanics, modifications, assists, the use of breath, bandhas and postural sequencing.

Art and Skill of Teaching: Expressed through our authenticity, sincerity, and willingness to be real. This means, removing any hint of "stage presence," or the need for approval. Simply, being as you teach. Letting love and joy move you in the class.

Your Own Personal Practice: Continue to develop your own practice, both for your own development and when necessary, to demonstrate the postures.

Professional Boundaries: This is one of the most important practices to be mindful of as a teacher. We demonstrate this by being centered and keeping a non-attached environment with students. If we feel a student "taking" energy from you, we need to stay within our integrity and silently say no. While each situation is different, we should do our best not to become "friends" with practitioners. This is a burden of teaching. This can compromise the class and instruction. This must be assessed and discerned on a case-by-case basis. The intention of this principle is to ensure we maintain a safe and neutral environment. It is not a black and white principle. Similar to leadership, as yoga teachers, a healthy distance should be utilized due to the energy dynamics that take place in a yoga class.

Surrender: This is one of the most effective ways to soften the ego and create an experience of humility. This understanding of humility aids in both self - healing and in holding space for others to do the same.

Ethical Guidelines for Yoga Instructors

Our most important responsibility is to set the example by the embodiment of personal integrity. We practice this through moral and ethical conduct, showcased by speaking unconditionally loving words, cultivating unconditionally loving thoughts and by engaging in unconditionally loving actions. Unconditional love is non-selective and free of judgment. We simply commit ourselves to this practice while knowing that we are human beings and will encounter difficulty. Continuously giving ourselves the same unconditional love and compassion that we strive to give to others, we actively nurture our growth towards truth, love, and joy.

General Ethical Considerations:

- Honor and love yourself. Be loving and gentle with yourself.
- Be genuine in a way that reflects your love and respect for yourself and others.
- Demonstrate humility. This is the understanding of your limitations. If you don't know, say, "I don't know." Be willing to research and bring an answer back with you.
- Show that a teacher is primarily a student. Let students know when they have taught you something new.
- Be modest. Do not try to impress your students. You are there to focus on them, not you.
- Welcome all practitioners, of all gender, race, religion, creed, nationality, cultural background or sexual preference.

- Give feedback by first observing what is right, what to celebrate – beauty, light, energy, in order to build confidence and remove doubt in practitioners. Just being on their mat is enough.

- Know yourself and seek self-improvement. Check your ego at the door. There is no room for a teacher's ego or projections in a class.

- Be polite, respect practitioners and address them by name when possible.

- Never physically or verbally demean or abuse a practitioner. You are there to create a safe and nurturing environment.

- Be compassionate and practice selfless service.

- Encourage and honor independent thinking, being, and exploring.

- Express that yoga is a process, never-ending, and all that is necessary is the will to practice.

- Be patient with yourself and students.

As with the practice of yoga, the principles and ethics of teaching must be practiced as well. A good gauge is to draw your awareness to the energy flowing within in you. Are you peaceful? Do you feel light? Or do you feel heavy? Ask those introspective questions daily, then write and reflect on what is taking place in your life to trigger such experiences of being. This path isn't always easy, but it is truly rewarding. Don't hesitate to ask for help and feedback through conversation, dialogue or connection. We are all here to nurture and support the growth of one another for this is the true act of love. [62]

Teaching Overview

When we first think of teaching yoga, the natural thought is the class itself. This is, of course, a huge part of teaching but it is not everything. Considerations for clothing, space, other teachers, props, music, etc. all go into creating an experience for students. My hope as a teacher is always that students walk away with a sense that teaching yoga

---

[62] The sections *Ground Rules, Developing as An Authentic Principle Based Yoga Instructor and Ethical Guidelines for Yoga Instructors*, was co-written by myself and my two other business partners, Melissa Love-Glidden and Ryan Krupa when we wrote our first Teacher Training manual in 2011.

must be easy. When everything flows well, the details are often overlooked by the average person. It is only when we as teachers struggle to make things work that it becomes obvious to students in our class. Below are some guidelines and considerations to prepare for all aspects of teaching a yoga class.

Clothing: As an instructor, you should dress in clothes that are comfortable for you to move freely allowing for the comfortable demonstration of poses. It is best to use your common sense to avoid any T-shirt slogans or advertisements that may be offensive. It is perfectly fine for you to have strong opinions about social or political issues for example, however teaching a public yoga class should not be the platform you choose for sharing these opinions. Pants that are too baggy may make it difficult to show leg position in poses. Too little clothing or too revealing clothing may make students uncomfortable. Understand your environment and your audience and use discernment.

Arrival: Arrive early to your class, so you have time to prepare yourself and your space. Take a moment to set up your mat and any props you will be using for demonstration. Prepare your space and be ready to greet students as they arrive. It may be helpful to arrive early enough to warm up your body through a light asana to avoid injury.

Before Class: As students enter the studio do your best to make them feel welcome and at home. Introduce yourself to new students and ask their name. Instruct them on where they can store their belongings as well as where the bathrooms are located. Inform them of any props they may need for class and ask to see if they have special considerations that should be taken into account during asana practice. Depending on your class size it may be necessary to help students set up their mats in a way that will be comfortable for all to move.

Preparing the Space: Create a sacred space for you and your students. The space should be clean and uncluttered. Position yourself in a space where you are visible to all students. Special consideration for music and aroma: Consider the fact that one person's music is another person's noise. Be conscious of volume and type. The right music at the right time can be a great addition to a class, but the opposite could also be true. For more on music, see the section titled: *What About the Tunes*. If you like to use incense, essential oils, or fragrant sprays, be considerate of the quantity and quality of the sources. Similar to music the right application can enhance the overall atmosphere and experience but too much can be distracting. Special consideration for essential oil or topical rubs should be made when considering individuals and possible allergies. Stick to simple ingredients and announce to your class what is in each. Give students an opportunity to let you know if they are allergic to an ingredient or would not like to have it sprayed or rubbed on their skin.

During Class: Focus on attuning the class. The first 10-20 minutes, the energies are attuning to one another. Focus on breath and easing everyone into the practice. Help build collective energy to create a shared experience while keeping it intimate and personal to each practitioner. Be observant and flexible. You are there to hold the energy of the room and to set the example for healing, not to command or control. Yoga is difficult, especially for beginners. Be supportive and encouraging. Keep your dialogue simple and concise. Don't talk all the time. Hold space for silence. Let students have their own experience, especially in the longer holds. Personal experience lands viscerally in students. It's a powerful way to connect and foster growth.

Moving into a pose
- Locate yourself where everyone can see you.
- Call the breath cue followed by the pose name, before further instruction. (example: inhale up to Warrior II)
- Name the pose in its English translation first. I tell new students, your first few classes are like playing Simon Says in a foreign language. They will have a hard-enough time with learning the poses in English. For more advanced classes you can work in the Sanskrit names if you'd like.

During the Pose
- Teach from the ground up. Foundation first.
- Be specific and use reference points to deepen the expression.
- Limit instructions to three or less cues at one time.
- Avoid negative language.

- Move with purpose. Pacing the room can be very distracting. Instead, scan the room to see poses from different angles and perspectives.

- Hold unilateral poses the same length of time on each side.

- Remind students to breathe.

- Work to avoid filer words (ok, good, beautiful, right). Positive feedback is encouraged but be mindful of your words.

- Saying a practitioner's name is powerful and supportive. Teach to individuals while moving the group energy.

- The pose begins when you want to come out of it.

Exiting the pose

- Synchronize the exiting movement with the breath (Exhale, plant your hands).

- Assess energy, breath, and attention of the students as they transition.

- Work resting poses into your flow if it seems appropriate.

<u>Ending Class:</u>

When class ends, assist your students with putting away any props and mats. Allow yourself to be present for questions and to see your students off. It is common for students to have questions after class and to make yourself available to them goes a long way. Be sure to clean the space before you leave. This may include mopping the floor, putting away props and removing your personal materials (mat, notebook, music, etc.)

Delivering the Message

It's not just what you say, but how you say it

Research has shown that communication is 55% body language, 38% tone of voice and only 7% the words you actually say. Posture, mannerisms and eye contact speaks volumes. A teacher's body can be an effective tool for emphasizing and clarifying the words you use while reinforcing your sincerity and enthusiasm.

It has been my experience that one of the biggest fears prospective teachers have is public glossophobia. More than 75% of people have this common fear of, yup you guessed it, public speaking. Don't worry. There are a few easy to practice techniques to help you overcome your fear.

Start Small: Start by only teaching a section of a full class to a small group of friends or family. This will give you an opportunity to begin to get comfortable with talking in front of people without overwhelming you with too much content and variables.

Prepare: Knowing the material will make you more comfortable. This means knowing your sequence and pose cues. This also includes practice. Walk yourself through your class on your mat or practice teaching your class just by saying it out loud.

Don't Memorize: You don't need to memorize a script. This can lead to an inauthentic tone and separate you from the class. Instead, do the proper preparation and allow any natural deviations to occur while teaching.

Use Your Breath and Visualization: The breath is a powerful tool to relax the body. Take a few slow deep breathes before you begin, or start off the class with some slow deep breathing that you participate in. Visualization is also a great tool. Before you teach, picture yourself leading the class with grace and confidence.

Find A Friend: A friend or familiar face can help to put you at ease. When first starting out ask for a friend to join you. If you start to feel nervous, focus on your friend. It will make you feel better knowing they are there, they support you, and they want you to be successful.

Channel the Energy: Stress can be your friend. Here's how it works. One of the responses your body has to stress is an elevated release of cortisol. While this hormone is necessary to cope with short-term stress physically, prolonged elevated levels of cortisol are associated with such things as impaired immune function and depression. When a stressful situation ends, your body has stress recovery hormones. Two of these hormones are DHEA and nerve growth factor. Both of which increase neuroplasticity which physiologically allows your brain to learn and grow from a stressful situation. The scientific term for this is stress inoculation. Higher levels of DHEA are connected to the reduced risk of anxiety, depression and more. The key is to have higher DHEA levels and lower cortisol levels. This elevated DHEA ratio to cortisol is called, the growth index of your stress response.[63]

Non-Verbal Communication

1. **Eye contact** establishes an immediate bond with practitioners, especially when a teacher focuses in on individual practitioner rather than just gazing over the class as a whole.

2. **Control mannerisms.** Mannerisms are the nervous expressions a teacher might not be aware of such as putting their hands in their pockets, nodding their head excessively, or using filler words like *um* and *ah* too often.

3. **Put verbs into action** when speaking to a class by physically acting them out with the hands, face or the entire body.

4. **Avoid insincere gestures** by matching facial expressions to the gestures being made by the body.

Verbal Communication

5. **Enunciate clearly.** Speak deliberately and clearly. Avoid the over use of Sanskrit words especially if you don't know how to pronounce them. Maintain a high level of vocal energy throughout your class. If you don't sound excited or enthusiastic about your class why would anyone else?[64]

6. **Speak at the correct speed.** Remember that you're leading a class through movement. That movement is more times than not matched with the breath. The human mind will move at speeds roughly four times faster than most people speak.[65] If you've already taught, you've probably experienced this. You're teaching a class, calling out the poses and sequence and suddenly you forget what the next move is. All you have to do is look around the room, and you will see bodies moving toward the next position. They are already thinking about it before you even say it. For this reason, speaking a little more quickly actually works to your advantage. Just like anything else, there is a balance to be found. Speaking

---

[63] (McGonigal, 2015)

[64] (Vassallo, 1990)

[65] (Vassallo, 1990)

like an auctioneer is distracting and impossible to follow. Speaking like Eeyore from Winnie the Pooh will have people dragging their limbs across their mats. Find the balance, increasing your speed slightly to keep up enthusiasm and movement.

7. **Be careful with tone.** Be confident with what you say. A common mistake of new teachers is to have the inflection in their voice rise at the end of a statement making it sound like a question. This puts doubt in the mind of the student and can disrupt your class. "Your voice is the instrument that you must use to convey your message. It has an infinite variety of pitch, level, and tones. You need to learn to play on it just as an accomplished musician coaxes inspired and beautiful sounds form a violin." – Wanda Vassalo

8. **Avoid slang and curse words.** Diverse classes may not understand certain slang terms thus losing their meaning and intent. Avoid the use of inappropriate language. While it may be quite common for you to say, it could be offensive to someone else.

What Not to Do

Chris Anderson is the head of TED talks. In his book on public speaking, he outlines four things you should never do in a TED talk. Since teaching group yoga classes is a public speaking forum, I've included three of the most relevant here.

The Sales Pitch: Many yoga teachers have second jobs or run other businesses. You should never use your class as a 60-90 minute sales pitch to get them to buy. Your job is to support, nurture and inspire when possible. You will learn later in the book that when you educate, inspire and teach; you never have to sell.

The Ramble: Leave space for silence. We are natural storytellers and a parable, myth or short story is a great way to communicate a moral, ethical or spiritual concept in a way that is interesting to your students but be careful. Keep it concise and to the point. You don't want to spend the first 20 minutes of your class rambling on without ever getting to your point. You also don't ever want to ramble about your own personal successes and achievements. Remember humility is a spiritual act.

The Inspiration Performance: Desikachar says in his book, *The Heart of Yoga*, "Yoga is different from dance or theatre. In yoga, we are not creating something for others to look at. As we perform the various asanas, we observe what we are doing and how we are doing it. . . if we do not pay attention to ourselves in our practice, then we cannot call it yoga." The same can be said for our teaching. We need to pay attention to what we're doing and why we're doing it. These are two philosophical questions that we should always be asking ourselves. What am I doing? Why am I doing it? A yoga teacher is there to hold a neutral space for practitioners to experience their own power through the tools of yoga. Do not put on a performance for students to see. You are there as a guide but not the main event.

What About the Tunes?

The Science of Music

The auditory system of the fetus is fully functional at about 20 weeks after conception. We are listening even before we are born. Newborns will recognize their parent's voice and can even show preference to a song they may have heard regularly in utero up to a year after birth.

Our brains are divided into four major lobes – the frontal, temporal, parietal and occipital – plus the cerebellum and brain stem. While the innerworkings of these lobes is quite sophisticated and integrated, each has been given generalized functions. The frontal lobe is responsible for planning and self-control. The temporal lobe works with hearing and memory. The parietal lobe works with motor movement. The occipital lobe works with vision, and the cerebellum is involved in emotions and movements. Music effects all four.

Because music has the ability to activate all areas of the brain, not only can it have us tapping our feet but it can bring up often repressed or discounted emotions within us, leading us to tears.

Remember the last scene of Gladiator? Lisa Gerard's voice draws us into the story, tugging on our emotions. Or what about Braveheart? The familiar tune of the bagpipes brings us back to the love and loss of William Wallace, championing us to his cause. When we are lying in Savasana at the end of a yoga class, and we hear those songs we are transported back to the emotional state that we first experienced them in. This has powerful consequences for the experience one might have in your class.

We are hard-wired to synchronize our bodies to move with the music. The human mirror neuron system can decode movement in melodies. An upward moving melody stimulates upward movement; "jumping for joy." A downward moving melody would have the opposite effect. Melodies can also be interpreted as speech. There is a melody tone in the human voice which can communicate feelings such as sadness, happiness, or boredom.

But how can we use this information to enhance the overall experience of our class?

The Art of Music in Class

A single peak or crown pose sequence starts with slower moving warm-up poses. It gradually increases in speed and intensity peaking around the end of our standing or balancing sequence, before turning back down towards forward folds, cool-down poses and eventually Savasana. Knowing what we do about the effects of music on the brain and emotions, we should do our best to match the melody and tempo of our music with the sections of our sequence.

For example. If I'm moving towards the peak of my sequence and have brought the class to the floor to do some core work (everyone's favorite thing to do!) I might choose music that has a steady and clear upbeat. The room needs to have energy and intensity to keep going. In an opposite fashion, once we reach Savasana, the melody should be one that can transport you to a relaxed and serene state.

Don't Over Do It

While music can be a great addition to any class, it can also have the opposite effect. The right music at the right time will enhance a student's overall experience, but the wrong music can ruin it. Use discretion and don't rely on music to carry the energy of the room but rather, enhance the experience. I personally like to teach a class without any music from time-to-time. Newer teachers can rely too heavily on their music and will learn a lot by teaching without it every so often.

Demonstration Principles

Demonstrating poses during your class can make it easier for students to understand what the pose looks like, especially if they are new. Below are the techniques that will help you demonstrate poses in a manner that clarifies a pose instead of making it more confusing.

Mirroring: If you stand to face your class when demonstrating, it is helpful for you to mirror them. What this means is if you are asking them to lift their left leg, for example, then you lift your right leg. Because we are such visual beings what we see has a tendency to override what we hear. We are also used to seeing the mirror image of ourselves reflected back to us. For some people mirroring comes easily. For others, it is much more difficult. If you are one, who has trouble with their left and right try this technique. On the top left corner of your mat write in a detectable marker the capital letter "R" for the right. In the top right corner of your mat write the capital letter "L." When you're mirroring, you can look at your mat to see which side you should call out.

Being seen: Whenever you demonstrate a pose you want to make yourself visible to as many of your students as possible. This way they don't have to come out of a pose or look around another practitioner to be able to see you. If you have the ability, you may try to stagger people's mats as the class is getting started. Doing this will set students up in a way that they are not directly behind the person in front of them. This will make it easier for them to see you at the front of the room when demonstrating a pose.

One step at a time: Some poses are difficult to describe and demonstrate at the same time. In these cases, take it step-by-step. Explain the pose first, and then demo, or demo first, and then explain it.

Use discretion: You don't need to demo every pose. Use your best judgment and be present with your class. Take notice if the entire room seems to be confused or only a select few. If it is only a select few, then you can approach them on their mat and offer a gentle assist or adjustment. It is challenging to take your own class and teach it at the same time. Anyone who has tried this has learned how quickly they can find themselves out of breath, making it hard to continue to call out the poses and the cues. Demonstrating every pose also leaves you stuck to your mat. This limits your ability to see the room and the students in it from different angles, which becomes very important when checking alignment and deciding if hands-on adjustments are needed.

Know your limits: There may be a pose that you feel would be helpful for the class, but you can't quite do it yourself. Make sure during your demonstration that you explain this. It may be helpful in these instances to refer them to look at someone in the class who can do the pose well. Humility is an important quality for a yoga teacher to embody. In this case, it connects you to your class and shows that you are also a student, right there with them.

Following these five principles will allow you to enhance your class and your practitioner's experience. As you practice teaching see how they can be applied and find the style that speaks most to you as an instructor.

Varying the Asana

There are two principle reasons to vary the asana. One is to expand one's physical capabilities, and two is to encourage attentiveness.[66]

Everyone comes to their mat from their own unique place and level of capability. Becoming aware of a student's capabilities, and adjusting the postures accordingly, is a skill that a teacher should practice. Yogasana should be balanced between stihra (steadiness) and sukha (ease). Varying a pose or poses, customizes a practice and allows for a student to find the balance between stihra and sukha with greater ease.

Practicing the same pose over and over can lead to boredom. As the body adjusts to a routine, it requires less mental effort to focus on the action. Remember, practicing the same sequence over and over again and, in the same way, can lead to a body that is going through the motions and a mind that is unfocused. Varying a posture or sequence can reinvigorate the mind to stay attentive.

Here are five ways to vary the asana

1. Varying the physical form. Example: Taking the ankles with Uttanasana, or softening the knees in Paschimottanasana.

---

[66](Desikachar, 1999)

2. Varying the breath. Example: Holding the breath for a moment at the top or bottom of a movement or leading the practice as one breath, one movement.

3. Varying the rhythm. Example: Breaking down the vinyasa into individual steps and then teaching it in a flow.

4. Adjusting the preparation. Example: Changing the preparatory postures. This can be used when building a class around a "crown pose."[67]

5. Adjusting the focus of attention. Example: Pulling the attention to the back foot in Humble Warrior.

Adjusting and Assisting

Assisting a student in a posture can be a very helpful act, giving practitioners a feeling of support, helping them create space and release while also stabilizing and deepening an asana. The right adjustment at the right time can help students deepen their expression of asana, advancing their pose and improving their experience. However, the wrong adjustment, at the wrong time, can have the opposite effect. It is your responsibility as an instructor to be mindful of your touch and deliver intentional helpful assists.

Your effectiveness as a teacher in doing this relies on your skills and knowledge in seeing, understanding and relating to practitioners in a meaningful, ethical and individualized way. The following section will increase your understanding of asana by cultivating a heightened sense of awareness of energy and anatomy, giving you both the knowledge and confidence to integrate hands-on adjustments into your classes.

The Science of Touch

The skin is composed of about 300 million cells, making it one of the largest organs in the human body. Within it are housed between six to ten million sensors conveying information about pressure, pain, heat, cold and tension. Some tell us we have an itch and others tell us we're hurt. Each one activates a different part of the brain, which in turn enables an emotional response (soothed, hurt, comfortable, distressed, angry or calm).

---

[67] A crown pose is a pose that is typically more challenging and/or more complex. A teacher builds up to this pose by preparing students with easier and less complex poses which use similar muscles groups.

Our sense of touch is the first sense to develop in the womb, as early as three weeks after conception and continues to refine throughout pregnancy. Some studies have shown that short bouts of touch (as little as fifteen minutes) enhance growth and weight gain in children and lead to emotional, physical, and cognitive improvements in adults.

Precise touch is shown to lower blood pressure, heart rate, and cortisol levels, stimulate the hippocampus (an area of the brain that is central to memory) and drive the release of a host of hormones and neuropeptides including oxytocin. Oxytocin is associated with the promotion of behaviors such as compassion and trust between individuals.

Research by Dr. Tiffany Field at the Touch Research Institute found that the brain is excellent at distinguishing an emotional touch from a similar, but non-emotional one. Her research identified that particular touch receptors exist solely to convey emotion to the brain not sensory information about the external environment. One experiment concluded that emotion could be conveyed through touch even when individuals were separated by a curtain. Furthermore, it was discovered that the emotions that are communicated by touch could go on to shape our behavior as mentioned earlier.

Dr. Field also compared the growth rates of premature infants who were maintained in incubators without touch (standard protocol) to those who were subjected to light massage several times a day. Babies in incubators are placed in a somewhat sterile environment, fed intravenously and often go for extended periods without touch. Both groups of babies were fed the same amount, yet the premature babies who were lightly massaged several times a day gained 21-47% more weight than the premature infants who were not touched.

Types of Touch

When making adjustments, the type of touch that you use will vary depending on the desired outcome. Here are a few different types of touch commonly used.

Investigative touch is used to check the quality of muscle or skin tension. This technique is useful in identifying if the proper muscles are active or inactive in a pose. Investigative touch will often be used at the beginning of an adjustment and then shift into directive touch.

Directive touch is probably the most common adjustment and is the application of firm contact which moves the body in a particular direction.

Alerting touch helps to bring a practitioner's awareness to a particular area. The teacher gently presses on a specific area without directing it to move. This gentle pressure is especially useful when accompanied by a verbal cue.

Sometimes in balancing postures, all a practitioner needs is some support to help them stabilize their position. **Supportive touch** can be used to stabilize their body giving them the freedom to explore the posture with more ease on their own.

With more restorative postures including many forward folds or supine poses, a **comforting touch** can be used to soothe and nurture. This type of touch can be very appreciated but should always be applied mindfully as it can easily be misinterpreted.

Adjustments should be offered after teachers have determined that they're necessary. **Unnecessary touch** with no particular reason or intention creates confusion and should be avoided. One particular type of unnecessary touch that should never be used is **angry touch.** This type of touch includes pushing, slapping, poking, grabbing, pulling, etc. If you are feeling angry, annoyed or frustrated in any way, it is best to avoid offering adjustments to anyone.

The Art of Adjusting
Before we can offer an adjustment, we need to have some basic understanding of how the body moves.

What is an adjustment? It is a small alteration or movement made to achieve a desired fit, appearance, or result. Why Offer an Adjustment? There are three reasons to offer a student an adjustment. They are: to move a practitioner deeper into a pose, back a practitioner out of a pose, and stabilize/support a practitioner in a pose.

A teacher should never press on an area of the body that is not supported by bone, such as eyes, throat and lower abdomen. Additionally, a teacher should never press at a joint but rather on the belly of the muscle surrounding a joint or another area of the body.

Moving a practitioner deeper into a pose means moving them deeper into one or multiple movement patterns. This movement usually involves increasing the amount of flexibility and strength required and decreasing the amount of contact they have with the ground. Backing a practitioner out of a pose works the exact opposite by decreasing the amount of strength and flexibility required while increasing the points of contact with the ground. Stabilizing a practitioner in a pose simply provides support to one or more areas of the body so practitioners can work with the pose themselves, to find their expression.

What if someone doesn't want to be adjusted?

There are numerous reasons why a practitioner may not want to be adjusted in class. They may include previous bad experiences, injury, past trauma or soreness. If a practitioner expresses a desire not to be adjusted, their request should be honored, regardless of their reason. There is no need for any further discussion. A teacher is there to serve practitioners to the best of his or her ability and honoring the request not to be touched, is part of that service. At MOSAIC our liability waiver states in bold that teachers may sometimes make hands-on adjustments and it is the practitioner's responsibility to let the teacher know if they do not want to be adjusted. It is recommended that you let practitioners know before class if you are planning to give adjustments, so they have an opportunity to let you know their wishes.

Adjusting Guidelines

"When you walk into class to teach, first connect with yourself. You cannot connect to your students if you are not in touch with yourself. Then connect to the student, the human being standing in front of you right now. Finally, connect to the task at hand, often an asana. Keep this order, and you will like what you say and do next. Teach from your wisdom with love and compassion". – Judith Lasater

Preparing to offer an adjustment consists of three steps; understand, observe, and choose. Each step is explained in more detail below.

A basic understanding of human anatomy including muscle groups and joints is important for offering effective hands-on adjustments. By understanding how different joints move and what muscles are responsible for that movement, you can maximize the efficiency of motion and avoid contraindications because the primary cautions will be known. It's also important to have an understanding of the pose itself. Different poses have different effects on the body. Standing poses challenge the body differently than balancing poses do. Understanding the pose and its effect will help you decide more specifically what adjustments to offer. Knowing the correct alignment for the pose gives you a rough template to assess and decide.

The more experience you have as a teacher, the more familiar you will become with common issues that practitioners have. This information allows you to pay close attention during poses or variations that you've come to find many practitioners struggle with.

I recommend that you maintain good hygiene practices. i.e., keeping your hands, feet, and body clean. It's usually best to keep your hands and feet fragrance-free. However, if you do choose to apply an essential oil, lotion, or other sports cream to your hands before making an adjustment, you should use caution and understand if there is anyone in your class that could have an allergy to one or more of the ingredients used.

The progression of a well-sequenced class moves the practitioner from a slower warm-up to a faster more intense peak and then back to a slower cool-down. This sequence structure gives you as a teacher the opportunity to begin to **observe** the physical capabilities of practitioners. You can learn a lot from observing Suryanamaskara A as it moves the body through flexion and extension of the legs, trunk, and arms. *Observing current physical capabilities is the second step towards deciding to offer an assist.* Next, you want to *observe the practitioner's breath and overall comfort level in the pose.* Every posture should be balanced between sthira and sukha. One of the first cues that a pose is out of balance is the breath. If the breath becomes short, labored, or cut off these are good indicators that a practitioner is pushing too hard into the body and should receive an adjustment or verbal cue to back out to a point at which they can breathe comfortably. Facial expressions and general tension in the body are other cues that the posture is not balanced. The clenching of the jaw, pained expression, exhausted expression, excessive redness in the face, etc. are all indicators of discomfort.

Once you have gathered all the previous information, step back and take a look at the general alignment of the pose. Does the pose look to be aligned correctly? Is effort being placed too heavily in one area or another? Take a moment to assess both the current state of the practitioner and the posture, then you're ready to move to the final stage of preparing.

Once you understand and observe, you are ready to make a choice. You should ask yourself two questions during this process. One, what is the purpose of the adjustment I'm going to give? Two, is there time to offer the adjustment before moving on with the class?

USING THE SUTRAS AS A GUIDE FOR HANDS ON ADJUSTMENTS

In the yoga sutras, Patanjali begins his eight-limb system with the five virtues that govern our relationships with others and the world. We can also use an understanding of these five virtues as a guide for ethically engaging others in hands-on adjustments.

Ahimsa – Non-harming: Through self-study, conscious intention and deliberate action we seek to offer assists that will help a practitioner deepen their expression of an asana without doing harm. The opposite of this is also true. We may look to provide an assist that backs a person out of an asana that their bodies may not be ready for so as to avoid injury.

Satya – Honesty: It is important that we are honest with ourselves about our ability and confidence in offering hands-on adjustments. As mentioned earlier we communicate with each other through touch. Being confident in your decision and ability instills confidence to the practitioner receiving the adjustment.

Asteya – Not taking what isn't yours: In this case, we're looking more at an experience. To apply Asteya in terms of adjusting, we want to be mindful of how we are altering a practitioner's experience of their practice. Sometimes it's ok to struggle a little as it helps us to learn and grow. As teachers, we need to be mindful of our intention and seek to subtly enhance or protect from injury, while allowing the overall experience to belong to the practitioner.

Brahmacharya – Acting in love and not selfishness: Traditionally this Yama relates to sexual restraint, but its essence can be applied here as well. It is important that you are clear mentally and emotionally before engaging physically with another person. If you find yourself engaged in romantic or lusting thoughts surrounding a practitioner, it is may be best not to offer an adjustment until you can be clear and supportive.

Aparigraha – Non-attachment: As you build your confidence and ability you may receive feedback that you offer "great assists." This in and of itself is a good thing but can boost one's ego leading to a feeling of having to offer adjustments even when they are not needed. Be confident in your abilities but also mindful of not getting attached to your skill and putting the practitioners needs first before your egos.

Making the Adjustment

Once you have gone through the three steps to prepare, you are ready to engage in making your adjustment.

When making a physical hands-on adjustment, move into a practitioner's space gradually. Rushing towards a person on their mat can be jarring and unsettling. Move with intention and clarity so as not to create confusion. Once you've entered their space, stabilize your posture first. Stabilizing yourself first is especially important when there are large size disparities between you and the person you are adjusting and in balancing postures. Once you are stable, stabilize the practitioner. Be mindful of the type, pressure, direction, and location of your touch. Make the adjustment gradually. Some teachers like to use an internal count to help them ease into an adjustment and ease out. For example, once touch has been initiated, you begin counting up to five. The adjustment peaks at five and then slowly releases out as you count back down to zero. The count can be increased or decreased depending on the adjustment. When adjusting balancing postures, it may be helpful to end with steady contact until it's clear that the practitioner has regained their balance and are ready for you to release.

The Four Cs of Adjusting

1. **Consideration**: This is the process of observing the practitioner and the situation. It includes considering a practitioner's physical capabilities and if there is time to make the adjustment without interrupting the rhythm of the class.

2. **Clarity**: Having absorbed all the information you need, you now need to ensure that there is a clear intention for your adjustment.

3. **Confidence**: Move into a practitioner's space with clarity and confidence. A student can sense if you are not confident with your adjustment and that will affect the overall experience. Be assertive, and strong, but also gentle and comforting.

4. **Control**: This includes stabilizing your body position first as well as applying slow and steady pressure. To apply pressure slowly keep a slow silent count from 0-5 as pressure increases. Hold as long as necessary and then start to release pressure from 5-0 until no longer making contact.

Other Types of Adjustments

Sometimes hands-on adjustments are not necessary. Here are some other techniques to help a person work with their practice.

Verbal

You may notice that multiple people are struggling with the same thing. In this case, offer a verbal cue to the entire class. Observe if your cue was effective in practitioners making corrections. If not, you may need to offer a verbal cue specifically to a particular student. You will have to discern if this cue is open to the class or more one-on-one. To make a one-on-one cue, position yourself next to the practitioner's mat and adjust your tone and volume directing the comment to them.

Energetic

Adjustments in this category fall under practices like healing touch. They are not focused as much on the physical position of the asana but more on adjusting the subtle energy of a practitioner. Eastern cultures have long-held belief in a subtle energy body that is interconnected with our physical bodies. Yoga uses asana and pranayama to move this subtle energy more efficiently through the body, clearing blockages and maximizing concentrations in the appropriate areas.

It is imperative with the energy modalities that you have clear and positive intentions before ever engaging in these types of adjustments. You should be grounded, aware and relaxed and use thoughtful non-sensual touch.

Sequencing

The Science of Sequencing
A 60-90 minute yogasana class takes practitioners on a journey through their bodies and minds. When properly sequenced, this journey has proven positive effects on both. Understanding both the science and art of sequencing is a valuable and important tool for any yoga instructor. Let's take a look at each of these categories, science and art, to deepen our understanding of what happens to a practitioner during their practice and how

to adjust variables to positively influence their experience.

Physiological Effects

The body is always working towards allostatic balance in attempts to optimize the performance of its many operating systems (digestive, cardiovascular, endocrine, muscular, etc.). The PNS and SNS systems are influenced by both physical and mental events both external and internal. In the case of yoga, some postures create internal physical stress through the external forces of gravity on the body in a given position. Our view on our ability to perform those poses may create internal mental stress if we see ourselves as "not being good enough" or "worse than others." Other poses, however, may create the opposite effect, relaxing the body and creating a state of mental relaxation and ease. Properly sequencing postures to create a harmony between these systems is an essential job of a yoga instructor.

The process by which we cope with stressors is called the alarm response. When there is a perceived stress, the body takes action. "Stressors" come in many different forms: an important deadline that needs to be met, an issue with a close relationship, a financial stress, or a difficult yoga pose. Anything that throws the system out of balance. When the stress comes in, an alarm goes off. The brain makes a decision on the severity of the stress and the appropriate response. If the subconscious decision to activate the sympathetic nervous system is triggered, a series of physiological events take place including:

- Increased heart rate
- Increased respiration
- Suppressed digestion
- Suppressed reproductive function
- Shunting of blood to the limbs
- The release of cortisol and epinephrine into the bloodstream

If you look at the list above, it sounds like all the things that can happen during a vinyasa class. This is because typical exercise routines place a stress on the physical body's homeostasis. If this stress is not dealt with and remains in place for a prolonged

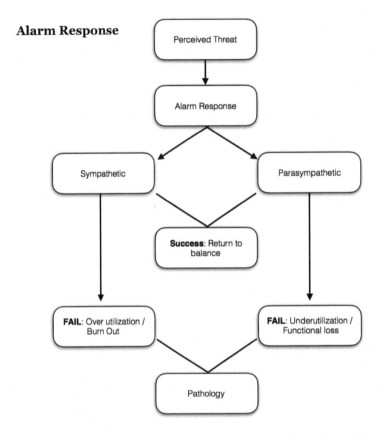

Alarm Response

period of time, it leads to system failure or burnout. On the other side of the scale, if the stress is not appropriately responded to, there is an underutilization of resources, often a lack of action (Tamas), and can also lead to pathology). ***The properly sequenced yoga class strengthens the nervous system, making it stronger and more resilient, and then allows for recovery back towards a parasympathetic state, avoiding system failures and pathology, with a focus instead on improving nervous system function.***

The peripheral nerves control conscious movement. Nerves extend from the spinal cord out to skeletal muscle tissue and through pathways of afferent and efferent nerves, which communicate information back and forth from our external environment to our brain and our brain back to our external environment.

Like any system in the body, if overworked, the nervous system can become fatigued. This is important to consider when learning new movement patterns.

When the body has repeated a movement pattern over and over again, it creates a program for it. Neural pathways in the brain are strengthened every time you repeat the pattern. In essence, neurons that fire together, wire together. As the neural pathways

172

strengthen, the action moves from a conscious area of the mind to a more subconscious area known as the basal ganglia. Think about how you can walk down the street and talk on the phone or send a text message at the same time. You don't need to think about every step you take. Your body knows how to walk without having to think about it. This frees your brain to perform other activities at the same time. It isn't until you step into the unexpected pothole that the movement pattern is then brought back up to the conscious level as it needs to adjust the pattern to the changing external environment.

When learning a new movement pattern, you don't yet have the neural pathways built to coordinate the movement, and so more effort and energy is required to complete the task.

Think of the first time you learned Warrior II. You had to pay close attention to the instructor's cues in order to align the body in the correct way. After a number of repetitions, you may have found that you transitioned into the pose with very little thought. You may even find yourself thinking about something else while in the pose. This is an example of how the mind is freed while performing a task that it has a motor pattern for. It is also an important reason for teachers to vary asana expressions.

Teaching Tip: For greater success teaching new movements, try to associate the movement with a pattern that may already exist. For example: associate chair pose with sitting back slowly not a bench

When teaching complex yogasana poses and movements, you should break down the movement into simpler parts first and then integrate them together. This makes it easier for the nervous system to assimilate the information properly.

A well sequenced class will start gradually to warm the body appropriately. There are two ways in which the body is warmed: extrinsic heat and intrinsic heat. Extrinsic heat comes from the outside environment, a hot yoga class for example. Intrinsic heat comes from the body's metabolism ramping up and creating heat as a byproduct of energy production. Warming the body from the inside out will improve muscle flexibility and reduce the likelihood of injury. Taking a "cold" muscle into a deep stretch without properly warming it up can lead to injury. The Sun Salutation series (Suryanamaskara A) in vinyasa yoga is a great series of postures used to warm the body and stretch the major

Sequence Intensity vs. PNS activation

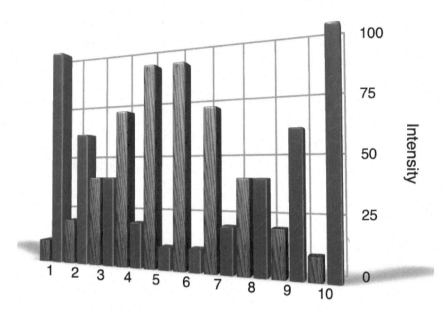

■ Intensity   ■ Parasympathetic activation

Pose Category

muscle groups throughout. This is why you often find this sequence taught at the very beginning of a class.

The Art of Sequencing

The art of sequencing a yoga class follows the science of how the nervous system works and the way in which the muscular system can be stretched to achieve healthy and safe gains in the postures. A common structure for a class is called the Arc Structure. This sequence builds a class on a bell curve beginning with simple movements and warm-up postures. The class progresses gradually as the pose selection becomes increasingly more difficult. This peak is usually around the halfway point of the class (30 minutes into a 60-minute class) and then begins to wind down, finishing again with some simpler movements and cool-down postures.

Arc Structure of Class

A 60-minute vinyasa class can be divided into approximately 10 different pose categories. They are as follows:

1. Seated meditation / pranayama

2. Warm-up

3. Suryanamaskara A

4. Standing Poses

5. Abdominals (optional)

6. Balancing poses (arm balances optional)

7. Backbending

8. Twists (can be worked into earlier categories as well)

9. Forward Folds

10. Cool-down (ending with Savasana)

You can see from the chart on the following page, how the arc structure of class works on the opposite curve of the parasympathetic nervous system. This sequencing style begins and returns a practitioner to a parasympathetic state, which aids in the body's ability to recover both physically and mentally from the practice.

1. Seated Meditation and Pranayama

This is an opportunity for practitioners to focus their minds, consciously allowing them to be on their mats and with their practice. It is an opportunity to set an intention for their practice or simply release their day up to that point. It is also a time to connect with their breath. Ujaii pranayama is a common breathing technique used throughout a vinyasa class, and it is at the beginning of class that an instructor has an opportunity to explain this technique. Other than seated, Child's Pose is a common posture used during this time.

2. Warm up

As mentioned earlier, warming the body slowly allows the muscles time to prepare for deeper stretches and works the nervous system through simpler movement patterns. Slower and simpler movements also allow a practitioner time to connect the mind, body, and breath together with more ease. This practice turns an asana practice into a yogasana practice. Yoga, meaning to yolk or unite, is enacted when the three separate parts of the practice become one conscious flow. The Sanskrit term for this is "vinyasa krama," or to move in a special and conscious way.

3. Suryanamaskara A

This sequence of postures created by Krishnamacharya flexes and contracts all the major muscles groups in the body. It has numerous variations that can be modified to adjust to both the level of the class or the ability level of the individual practitioner. This flowing sequence has also been shown to increase heart rate and when weaved in throughout the practice can have positive effects on the cardiovascular system.[68]

4. Standing Poses

Standing poses can be divided into two categories: neutrally rotated (Crescent Warrior or Warrior I for example) and externally rotated (Warrior II or Triangle pose for example). Generally speaking, neutrally rotated poses are practiced first, as they coincide most closely with static postural alignment and relate well to poses that transition gradually from the warm-up. Externally rotated poses can be more challenging, as they are not often a common position for the body to be held so require more attention in proper alignment. Practicing these categories in groups is best to help progress a practitioner deeper from pose to pose. For example Sequencing Warrior II -> Extended Side Angle -> Triangle, continuously opens the hips while leaving other alignment points in the same position.

5. Abdominals

Core activation is an essential part of any movement. It is from our core that movement patterns are first learned. When we were infants, we began to move our limbs from what is called a naval radiation pattern. Both our head and tail (sacrum) were as much limbs as

---

[68] It should be noted that the overall cardiovascular conditioning in yogasana in minimal when compared to other exercise activities like swimming, running, cycling, and other team sports where there is a noticeable strain on respiration and cardio output.

our arms and legs. Movement originated from the core and extended out to the limbs. In this way, we strengthened our core as well as the musculature around the spine, which gave us the strength to lift our head, push-up, crawl, and eventually walk. Of the core muscles, there should be a particular focus on the transverse abdominals. This is the deepest layer of the core muscles which help to stabilize the lumbar spine. Keeping the transverse abs engaged during many standing and balancing poses supports the back, making the pose more stable and safe. This is why abdominals are placed before balancing poses. By working the abs in a gradual and more focused way, we awaken them from the subconscious to the conscious level. This core-awakening will make our balancing poses more stable and easier to achieve.

6. Balancing Poses

Balancing poses can occur any time one foot is lifted from the ground, as in Warrior III, or one hand is lifted from the ground, as in Side Plank, or we are inverted and balancing on our hands/arms. Challenging the balance challenges the nervous system and can make us more stable in our everyday living, strengthening our righting reactions. It also improves our dynamic stability.[69]

7. Backbending Poses

Poses in this category extend the spine, strengthening the muscles along both the back plane and the front plane of the body. Backbending postures are a good counter to the possible crunching movements of abdominal exercises. The cervical and lumbar spines extend deeper than the thoracic spine does. The opposite is then true for forward folds. Careful consideration should be taken when backbending that the spine is lengthened and supported by the core musculature to avoid any pinching or pain in the lower back. The Valsalva maneuver is commonly described as a technique to achieve this. To perform, simply draw the bellybutton up and in towards the spine to engage the transverse abdominals. This activation will help keep space between the vertebrae of the lumbar spine as well as control the movement.

---

[69] Righting reactions are typically built into the nervous system by the age of three and are responsible for keeping the head in a normal position, righting the body to a normal position, and adjusting the body parts in relation to the head.

8. Twists

Part of a well-sequenced asana practice is moving the spine in all directions, which means moving it on all planes. This translates to flexion/extension, lateral flexion/extension, and rotation. When we twist the spine, we are rotating it along the transverse axis. Twisting postures can be integrated into standing poses, as in Twisted Crescent Warrior. Using the breath is important for carefully guiding a practitioner into a twist. The inhales lift and lengthen the spine as well as open the ribcage while the exhales allow room in the abdominal cavity to move deeper into a twist. Simply practicing twisting deeper into a pose while taking an inhale breath makes this obvious. Other than standing postures, twists can also be integrated into seated poses and then become applicable to both the warm-up and cool-down categories of a sequence. Simple seated twists help prepare the spine for more challenging expressions and can also slow down the body and breath before Savasana.

9. Forward Folds

Forward folds are a good counter to backbending. Forward folds are more grounding. When performed seated, they are an opportunity to slow down the breath and heart rate. Forward folds work the spine into flexion and stretch the muscles of the back. They also help practitioners learn how to use the breath in a more controlled way. When we move into a deep forward fold, it becomes more difficult to take a deep breath. The ribcage and abdomen are constricted, forcing the breath into the back of the body. Exploring the practice of breathing into the back can help with future pranayama practices.

10. Cool-down / Savasana

The cool-down category consists of a number of different poses from multiple categories (backbends, inversions, twists). It is the way these poses are performed which establishes them as a cool-down. Generally speaking, cool-down poses involve the body having more contact with the floor and require little flexibility and little strength to perform. Some of the positions of the poses can also assist in shifting the body to more of a parasympathetic-dominant state, bringing the practitioner back to balance.

For example, you can take a Supported Bridge position with a block under the sacrum. This elevates the heart higher than the head, triggering the baroreceptors in the arterial wall to lower heart rate and blood pressure. The block allows for a release of muscular effort in the gluteus muscles as well as the lower back and quadriceps. In contrast, without a block, this pose can become more challenging.

The cool-down category ends with the final posture of our sequence, Savasana or Corpse Pose. In this position, the muscles relax, and the breath comes back to a natural rhythm. Savasana is an opportunity for practitioners' bodies and minds to absorb the benefits of their yoga practice and to take the seat of the passive observer. In Corpse Pose, we become the witness to the breath, body, and mind by simply remaining still and observing everything that's going on in our bodies and mind with a healthy detachment. The name of the pose also implies a reflection upon the impermanence of the body and all things of form. Eventually, the body will die. Corpse Pose gives us an opportunity to connect with the "Atman" or Soul inside of us that will remain on into the next life.

Sequencing across Categories

Many poses maintain a very similar shape in the body but rotate its position in space to create a new expression.

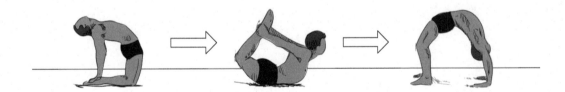

sequencing across pose cateogories

This is valuable information for a yoga teacher when looking back at the science of learning movement. You can help teach students new poses by relating the new pose to ones they already know from another sequence category.

179

Think about other poses in your practice that could be cross-category poses. Consider if you were to hold the position of the body but rotate the axis off of one point. What other posture might it become?

Personal Observances and Teaching Points

Begin where you are

The only place we can begin is exactly where we are. It is our job to accept this and move mindfully from this understanding.

Forcing yourself into a pose or poses because you see someone on your Instagram feed doing it, but knowing full well that your body is not capable or ready, is not a smart move. Your practice should be a dialogue. You direct the position and then listen to the feedback. I teach that there should be at least three breaths to a pose. The first breath is the habit pattern. It's where you go because you've been there before. The second breath is an opportunity to feel and receive the information from your body and mind about your current state. The third breath is the time to then mindfully adjust the position. This is the same concept that Iyengar has been quoted as referring to when he says, "pose and repose." While yogasana is a physical practice, yoga is a practice for the mind as well. We use the discipline of asana to inform the discipline of our life. If we push our bodies to a place they are not ready to go, we are moving from our ego. In yoga, the ego is seen as an obstacle that contributes to the ignorance of our true nature. Supporting its development with asana is counterproductive.

How do you know when you're moving from your ego? In Father Richard Rohrs book, *Immortal Diamond*, he says, "The ego always has an opportunistic agenda. The soul has no agenda whatsoever except to see what is-as it is- and let it teach you." When you are practicing yoga, you are moving from soul when you release your agenda and allow yourself to be fully immersed in the experience of the moment. It is in those moments on your mat when you shift to a more awakened state of being.

When teaching, do your best to observe where practitioners are throughout the class, offering options to deepen a pose or make it easier while encouraging them to find their individual boundaries in a non-competitive or aggressive way. I like to make a point to highlight a student in class not only when they take a new more advanced position but also when they honor their body and limits and modify the pose to make it less advanced and more appropriate for their current level of ability.

Breath is Your Teacher

TKV Desikachar says in his book, *The Heart of Yoga*, "Your breath should be your teacher." He goes on to explain that throughout your yoga practice, your breath should never become overly labored. Unlike many other exercises where deep, heavy breathing lets you know you're working hard, in your asana practice, the breath should be under control and easily flow in and out. A common pranayama technique for vinyasa is ujjayi breathing. With the lips closed, the tongue on the roof of the mouth, and a slight constriction of the glottis in the throat, the breath takes on an audible sound similar to that of an ocean wave as it rolls up onto a sandy beach. Additionally, the breath takes on a texture. Paying attention to both the sound and texture of the breath as well as the tempo, depth, and relative ease can help us realize when we are pushing too hard or attempting a pose that the body is not ready for. If you've been practicing asana for a while, you have probably experienced an arm bind or twist where there was a noticeable constriction of the breath. This, according to Desikachar, would be an indication that you should use a strap, take a half bind, or maybe no bind at all until you are able to complete the movement without constricting your breathing. Again, it challenges our ego to practice in this way.

Observe practitioners in class. If you notice that someone is having difficulty with the breath, suggest that they release their ujjayi breathing for a little while or give a modification to help adjust the pose to a level that fits the practitioner's capabilities.

Warm-up the whole body

This was mentioned earlier when discussing the science of sequencing but is worth noting again. Warming up the body helps to prepare the joints, muscles, heart, lungs, and mind. In a well thought-out sequence, you will work with every major muscle group and joint in the body, so preparing them is important. Warming the body will help to reduce the risk of injury as well.

Pose & Counter pose

Yoga is a practice that teaches balance. If we are to apply the philosophy to the asana, then you need to keep balance in the body. Specifically, you should be mindful of counterposes. A counter pose is a pose that works the body in the opposite direction of the pose before it. An example might be Camel Pose to Plow Pose. One is a deep backbend (extending the spine). The other being a deep forward fold (flexing the spine). In between, we bring the spine back to neutral to avoid the risk of injury.

Be sure to work counterposes into your sequence. Some key points when counterposing:

- Bring the joints back to neutral first.
- Counter poses should be easier than their opposite.
- Hold the pose and counterpose for even amounts of time.

Rest

Not everyone comes to their mat at the same level physically, mentally, or emotionally. You have to pay close attention to the tempo, temperature, and intensity, making sure to work in opportunities for rest. If you begin to see multiple practitioners dropping into Childs Pose, this is a good indicator that there are even more people in the class who would appreciate the break and who probably need it. Assess the energy in the room, facial expressions, exasperated noises, and breathing patterns. It is important that practitioners have an option to rest and recover if needed.

If we follow the arc structure of a class, a good time for rest is just after the peak of intensity. This rest can come in the form of Childs Pose or even standing in Mountain Pose. Anything that puts the body at relative ease and allows for a few deep breaths, toweling off sweat, and/or a quick water break will really help.

Outside Influences

As human beings, we are part of nature. We are connected to the environment around us in a very intimate way. The changing seasons, times of day, temperature, the cycle of the moon, location, air quality, and many other factors all influence now we feel when we step on our mat for practice.

For this reason, outside influences should be considered when organizing a sequence. Let's look at how they affect a class.

An early morning practice finds you on your mat after the body has been at rest for ideally eight or more hours. The muscles will be noticeably more stiff and possibly the mind a bit sleepy. For this reason, the pose selection and sequence at large should focus on a slow and extended warm-up series to awaken both mind and body. Some pranayama might be done to help focus the mind before asana practice.

In contrast, an early evening class finds us on our mat after a day of movement. The body will be noticeably more open and ready to move than in the morning, but the mind may be more fatigued, depending on our day. Cortisol levels are on the decline, and late evening practice may occur after dinner. It is advised that you not stuff yourself with food before any practice, but as a teacher, do bear in mind that some students may have just eaten. Inversions and twists may need to be adjusted or avoided. In opposite fashion to an early morning practice, more focus should be placed on the end of practice cool-down. Depending on how late the practice is, it may be some of the final activity a person will do before preparing for bed. That being the case, you will want to do your best to leave them in a parasympathetic state ready to rest and relax for the remainder of the evening.

The seasons affect both temperature and mood. Seasonal Effective Disorder is a condition in which a person experiences symptoms of depression based on the weather/season. The winter months in many areas of the country are much colder than the summer. Depending on where you're practicing, you may need to prepare the room to provide a comfortable temperature for practice. The days are also shorter. Energetically it is a time of withdrawal. Like the trees going dormant for the winter, people may display the energy of dormancy. Using the asana to bring a healthy balance to this while still honoring it is a good idea.

In the summer, days are longer and hotter. Energetically it is a time of opening after the spring of new birth and beginnings. Energy may be higher and more outwardly expressive. Again, using the asana practice to honor this while balancing it is worth consideration when composing your sequences.

Finally, a consideration of location. Practice on the beach in Hawaii might be put together a little differently than a practice in a renovated urban loft in downtown New York.

A well-sequenced yogasana class leaves a practitioner with a feeling of accomplishment and ease. There are many factors that go into the composition of such a class, that when mastered improve the overall experience for students in mind, body, and spirit.

Mindfully segment your class

10-15 minutes:	Opening meditation, pranayama & warm-up, Sun A & B
20-30 minutes:	Standing postures, abdominals, balancing
5-10 minutes:	Backbends, arm balances
5-10 minutes:	Forward folds, gentle inversions, floor
5-10 minutes:	Savasana

Yoga: The Business

You may be thinking about starting your own yoga studio, or maybe you would like to add a service to an existing practice.   Whatever the reason or interest, the following information will cover some of the basic principles for creating and marketing your business.

When people think of running their own business, they can be blinded by the "glamour effect." They instantly sink into thoughts of making their own schedule, doing what they love, practicing yoga all day and taking three vacations a year. These are all possibilities, but make sure you set realistic expectations is important.

Running a small business means that you are the CEO, bookkeeper, marketing manager, front desk staff, administrative personal, etc. You do pretty much everything! You need to be ready for a large time commitment. You also need to be ready to work through setbacks. It might not be smooth sailing the entire way so when the going gets tough, you have to practice persistence. If it's something, you are truly passionate about, don't let anything stop you from being successful.

The best thing you can do to prepare for starting a new business is to sit down and write a business plan. There are numerous templates, models, and services available to aid you with this. Writing a business plan will help you iron out all of the details discussed below as well as many others.

Starting Out

One of the first things a newborn gets after birth is a name. Seems fitting that a new business gets the same thing. In many ways, it will be like a baby to you for a while. So, what are you going to call your business? You want to pick something that helps to simply communicate something about who you are and what you stand for. Our studio is named MOSAIC. We created it to bring together people from all different backgrounds, beliefs, colors, nationalities religions, etc. Like individual pieces of a tile mosaic, each person has their own unique characteristics and beauty. You can also bring the pieces together to create a larger piece of art. Choosing a name is not a process that should be rushed. You want to make sure you are very happy with it. I would suggest sitting with the name for a while before finalizing anything. The last thing you want to do is create all of your marketing materials and then decide you want to change the name.

Some questions to ask when thinking of a name

- What is my mission?
- What type/style of yoga do I offer?
- Does anyone else already have this name? (Especially important when registering a business entity)
- What do I want my name to "say" about my business?

Registering your business entity

After you have your name, you will need to decide what type of business entity you will want to be. Different entities have different benefits. Below is a high-level overview of some of the popular business entity options.

- Sole Proprietorship: This is the fastest and easiest business structure to create. In most states, you will have to head down to your town hall building, fill out a form and pay a small registration fee. If you're going to be doing business by another name (referred to as a DBA or Doing Business As), you will indicate the name on this form. Once the name has been approved, you're all set. You will then be able to open a bank account in your businesses name.

- LLC (Limited Liability Company): A limited liability company might be your best choice if you are going into business with other partners, sometimes referred to as managing members. You can indicate the percentage ownership and the roles of each member. An LLC allows for a few ways to handle the business money as well. You can keep the company earnings separate or do something called pass-through taxation, passing them on to the managing members. LLC also gives you an extra layer of liability protection. If for some reason, you were to find yourself in a lawsuit, the assets of the business remain separate from those of the owners. This means your personal assets would not be subject to being taken, only the business's assets are. With a sole proprietorship, this is not the case.
- S – Corp: S-Corporations are set up similar to LLCs in some ways. One difference is that an S-Corp stands as its own entity. It will then be taxed as such. There is no pass-through taxation like there is with an LLC.

Before making a decision do your research on each entity and see which one will best fit you and your business before moving forward.

Operating Your Business

Here are examples of the different departments common to a yoga studio. Each department handles different tasks. If entering into a business partnership you should clearly outline all departments, tasks, and who is responsible for handling them.

Accounting

Don't forget about the money; someone has to manage it. Open a bank account in your business's name. Keep your personal money and the business money separate. This will help you track your business expenses and have a clearer understanding of your business' financial situation.

If you have the means financially to find a bookkeeper to track sales, receipts, expenses, and help you stay on your budget, that is great! For many small business owners, however, this is a service that is more a luxury than a necessity. If that's you, then you will need to keep the books yourself. Purchase an accounting software like Quickbooks or Quicken to help keep you on track. Do your best to reconcile your books monthly. Ultimately, it's a lot easier to go back over the bank statements for one month to find errors then it is to go back over 12.

Human Resources: Hiring & Firing, Customer Service, and Public Relations

Studio Maintenance: Cleaning, Supplies, Technical Support, Maintenance, Client Accounts, and Props

Information Technology IT: Website maintenance, Mobile App, Client Software, Phones, and Computers

Marketing Your Business

The key to any service businesses success is to get new people through the door and then to retain them. That's it! Here's how you do it.

Down to the Basics

Before crafting a major marketing plan, you need to have something to market and a way to communicate. Developing brand colors, a logo and mission statement are key. You want to make something simple, recognizable and consistent.

Register your web domain and build a website. Your website should keep consistent with your logo and brand colors. On your website, you will have a platform to deliver a little more about who you are and what services you offer. When first creating your website you should register your site with major search engines as well, to improve your visibility.

Everyone uses social media. Once you have your logo, brand colors, and website up and registered, you can create your social media pages. I would suggest that you start simple and build up. Unless you're able to hire a full-time marketing position, it's better to be consistent on a few key platforms than to be sporadic on a ton. When deciding which social media platforms to use, consider where your target audience would be most likely to see you. This leads us to the next step. Who is your target audience?

Your Ideal Client

Classes – General Public	Yoga Teacher Training
Personal fulfillment:	Personal fulfillment:
Value to Marketplace:	Value to Marketplace:
Profits:	Profits:
Total Score:	Total Score:
Private Classes	**Workshops**
Personal fulfillment:	Personal fulfillment:
Value to Marketplace:	Value to Marketplace:
Profits:	Profits:
Total Score:	Total Score:

Within the yoga industry, there are many subcategories. For example, you could be a teacher of public classes or private clients. You can host Yoga Teacher Trainings or shorter workshops. When deciding on your message, you should first decide where you want to focus your efforts. This doesn't mean you only communicate to one category, but it helps you navigate the level of effort in each one. Additionally, each category may have a different target audience. Below is a chart adapted from *The One Page Marketing Book*, by Alan Dib. In each box put a number between one and ten next to each of the three parts of the category (personal fulfillment, value to marketplace and profits). One being the lowest and ten the highest. Then add up each individual category to get an idea of where you would like to focus your efforts. I've included four common categories for yoga studios, but you can change them to whatever works best for you and your business

Aim small, miss small. When crafting your message, you need to know who it's intended for. The clearer you get on who you want to be teaching, the easier it will be to find them. To understand your desired audience you need to find your niche. Start first with your "market." In this case that's yoga. Then identify your "sub-market." Maybe that's teacher training. Then find you niche. Let's say you are going to lead trainings specifically on anatomy. If you can find a niche that nobody else is working in than you are in a great place! This is what marketers call a "blue ocean," because you don't have any competition (sharks) fighting for the same clients (fish).

A common technique to establish clarity of your target audience is to create an avatar. An avatar is a fictional person that you assign as many characteristics to as possible (age, gender, interests, needs, work, education, hobbies, etc.) The further you develop this avatar the better you start to understand them. Where do they like to shop? What type of music do they listen to? What social media channels are they on. How do they like to spend their recreational time, and most importantly, what is their biggest pain and how do you solve it?

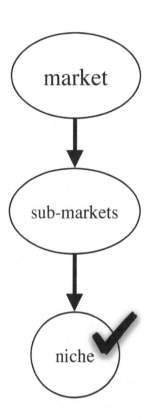

The Four Types of Customers

In *The One Page Marketing Plan*, Alan Dib outlines four different types of customers. I can't tell you how many "ah-ha" moments went through my head as I read this list.

1. The Tribe: Ideal fans and supporters of your business (This is who you want!)

2. The Churners: Come in on an aggressive deal or marketing campaign and really cannot afford you. When they realize this, they churn out and can be bad PR for your business back in your market.

3. The Vampires: They can afford you, but you can't afford them. They consume massive amounts of time and resources for the same price as everyone else. They want to talk to the owner and wants the owner to adjust everything more to suit them. They suck the blood out of your business.

4. The Snow Leopard: Exquisite and beautiful but rare and almost impossible to replicate. They are fun to work with, and the team and leaders love to spend time with them. Overall they're a bad investment because of their rarity, so are not good for a growth strategy.[70]

---

[70] (Dib, 2016)

When starting a new business, it's easy to think that every customer is the ideal customer, especially when we think in the simple terms of each customer = money, and I need money to survive. Of course, the principle is true, a business does need money, but it also needs to evolve and the best businesses don't survive, they thrive. Placing too much energy and effort in the churners, vampires, and snow leopards is going to leave you exhausted and eventually will damage your business's financial health and reputation. This is why you need to build a tribe. The one question you are always asking yourself is what are my tribe's primary pains and how do I alleviate them?

What is a Tribe and Why is it Important?

A tribe is a group of people that share two qualities: a shared interest and a way to communicate.[71] Tribes are led by leaders not managers. Managers streamline existing processes to make an outcome that is easier and less expensive. Leaders inspire change by turning a shared interest into a passionate goal. When a tribe is strong and inspired it leads to a movement. Think about the company Apple with Steve Jobs. He took a flailing company and turned it into a tribe of passionate members looking to the future of technology.

Your yoga business (or any business for that matter) will be strong if you can properly identify the correct candidates to be a part of your tribe, inspire them, and give them a platform to contribute and share with you and each other.

How Do I Build a Tribe?

Tribes don't just complete a task they create a movement, so the question you then need to ask yourself is, how do I create a movement? Russell Brunson, author of *Expert Secrets*, gives us three key elements needed to create a movement.

1. A Charismatic Leader – Movements are led by a charismatic leader. Charismatic leaders live a life that their tribe members admire. They have clear flaws but have overcome them to strengthen their character and grow. A charismatic leader maintains absolute certainty about their mission. No matter what the outside challenge the leader shows persistence and faith in the cause. A charismatic

---

[71] (Godin, 2008)

leader is able to walk the line between mainstream and crazy, which makes them interesting.

2. A Cause – Your tribe needs someplace to put their hopes and faith and its not the status quo. That is why a cause needs to be future based. This means your cause creates a vision for the future that your tribe can rally behind and get excited about. You as their leader need to help them do this. Part of rallying your tribe is to allow them to self-identify with the cause. This goes back to the avatar you created earlier. If you understand your tribe, you understand their wants and desires, as well as their pain. They need to be able to connect with your movement. One way to do this is to create an ethos. Here is the ethos that I created for MOSAIC. You may remember this from the beginning of the book.

A MOSAIC yogi is the **next generation of yoga**.

Strong, focused, loving, disciplined and **FREE.**

MOSAIC yogis **embrace** both flesh and spirit, reason and faith, technology and indigenous wisdom, East and West.

MOSAIC yogis use their resources to **alleviate the pain** and suffering of others.

MOSAIC yogis do not practice in front of a mirror because their practice is the mirror. They are **fearless in uncovering their** truth regardless of what they find.

MOSAIC yogis put **ethics and value**s before vanity and glory. They work harder, train harder and give more on and off the mat.

MOSAIC yogis use the asana practice not only to **build strength and flexibility** in their body but also in their mind.

MOSAIC yogis strive to recognize the divine light in all beings and treat each individual with **respect and love**.

MOSAIC yogis have been tired, injured, broken and lost but they **always find their way** back to their mat.

MOSAIC yogis practice with a **peaceful heart and a warrior spirit**.

MOSAIC Yogis
Are **One** Family

Have **One** Focus

Create **One** Future

To *Awaken and Uplift*

3. A new opportunity – Movements aren't generally created by improving upon an existing idea or product. Peter Thiel wrote an entire book on this one subject titled *Zero to One: Notes on Startups, or How to Build the Future*. In this book he talks about a number of different start-up companies that created a movement not by improving on something already in existence but by creating something entirely new. A prime example is of this is Facebook. Facebook paved the way for a whole category of connecting. Many companies have come after it to improve upon or tweak the focus but Facebook was the original giant. If you can think of a new opportunity within your field of expertise, be a charismatic leader and rally a cause you will have a tribe ready to follow.

Crafting your message

The marketing term for this is a Unique Selling Proposition or USP. Your USP is the primary reason that your clients should buy from you and not your competition. Here is an example of a USP that I created for my studio, MOSAIC.

MOSAIC offers a unique experience merging the traditional values and philosophies of yoga with the modern-day lifestyle. We use the asana to strengthen the body, steady the mind and cultivate benevolence of the spirit. We do not cut the soul out of the practice but make it very much a part of the journey.

We treat our tribe like family. Our instructors will know you by name and are willing to take extra time to answer your questions and help you grow not just on the mat but off of it.

We provide an environment that is supportive yet challenging. We teach upon the mat beside you as spiritual warriors together dedicated to awakening to our highest truth and to uplifting our soul and the souls of others.

Creating your own USP will help you to better craft your message and easily explain to potential clients who you are, what you do and why they should practice with you. But how do you get them to even talk to you?

Capturing Leads

Leads are potential clients that have not yet purchased your service. They can be acquired through a number of different channels. It is recommended that a business not have a "single point of failure." Meaning, you should not have one source of leads, one major customer, or on one type of media. This makes your business fragile and drastically limits your new lead potential.

Some leads can be generated with no cost while others are acquired through advertising and promotional dollars. It is important that "budget" not be set to restrict efforts that work. This is essential because if the ROI (return on investment) is positive, the budget is endless. For example, if you make $10 on every $5 spent there is no limit to the budget because it consistently produces a profit. Below are some key terms used in marketing to classify and leads and advertising efforts.

- Response rate = Total volume sent divided by number of people who respond
- Closure rate = Total volume sent divided by number of people who purchase
- **Customer acquisition cost*** = Cost of campaign ÷ clients acquired ($100 campaign / 2 customers acquired = $50 acquisition cost. If sale exceeds $50 winning campaign)
- ROI (Return On Investment) = Amount of $ earned from invested advertising dollars
- Front end = Money made up front on a campaign
- Back end = Money made after the initial sale. (Another term for this is Retention)
- Lifetime value = Front end + back end

*Most important number in advertising

There are lots of ways that new leads can be captured. Think creatively about your ideal client and where you might be able to grab their attention. Below is a list of some possible lead capture sources.

1. Referral from existing clients: the more of these, the better.

2. Social media advertising: find the correct channels. Where do you clients hang out and talk?

3. Website email automation: Offer a free e-book or online class in exchange for an email address.

4. Joint Ventures: find a similar but not identical business and create a partnership of referrals.

Nurturing Leads

It is a common mistake of most small business owners to think that you only need to contact potential clients a few times. Some research suggests that a person needs to be contacted as many as 12 times before they make a decision .[72] This doesn't mean that you flood their inbox with a sales pitch every day, or that you call them and beg them to come in for a class. You want to make sure that you are a welcome guest and not a pest.

You'll Never Have to "Sell" Again

When it comes to sales, you should stop thinking about selling something. Seems counter-intuitive but it's true. Instead, you need to position yourself as an expert in your field. Instead of selling, you are establishing yourself as a leader in your field by educating and advising. Your content and messaging needs to add value. Leaders create content; followers consume it. Good leaders are prolific content creators.

Send out a newsletter with the latest research on the health benefits of yoga, or post a video on how to safely get into shoulder stand. These are just a couple examples of how you can stay on your potential client's radar without forcing a sales pitch on them. Nobody likes that.

A few other techniques for making sales easier are as follows. One, keep the process simple. Eliminate any part of the process that could stop someone or make it challenging to complete the sale. The more streamlined, the better. Two, limit the options. Too many options make for confusion and confusion leads to delay in sales or no sale at all. Instead of 10 different class pass options try three to five.

---

[72] Dib, 2016

Everyone who is reading this knows that yoga is good for you. Whether you are a yoga teacher currently or want to become one in the future, chances are you want to share with others the benefits that you've experienced in your own life through your practice. This is a noble endeavor and one you should be passionate about. The second a client walks through the door you should be doing your best to deliver a world class service. This includes making them comfortable in the space, teaching the best class imaginable and helping them in any way they need. Teaching yoga is a service-based industry, and you should always be striving to serve better than they have ever experienced in the past.

Generating Referrals

Referrals are probably the most influential marketing tools a business can have. Someone is considerably more likely to try out a class when asked by a friend or family member then they are when prompted by an advertisement or flyer. Why? Trust! We trust the people close to us to have our best interest at heart. Even beyond that, we might do something with a friend just because we care about them and want to share in something that's important to them.

When asking for referrals, you should determine who you're asking and what type of referral you want. Be specific. Are you looking for a referral to your teacher training program or to try out your new student promotion?

Overall the equation is pretty simple. Communicate to your ideal client (tribe member) using your USP. Let them know how your service solves their problem. You can achieve this through many different channels, but if you're spending money to do it, then you want to have a positive ROI. Once your new customer comes to take your class, workshop or training deliver a stellar service so that they come back and become a raving fan and are more than happy to refer their friends and family to you. Here are a few examples of ways to generate referrals

• Use a software platform that awards points to current customers for referrals. Once you have this make it easy. Place a referral button on your monthly newsletter or social media pages

- Directly email potential clients for bigger ticket items like your teacher training program. Reach out to past participants and ask them to connect you with anyone they think would benefit from the program.

- Offer account credit to anyone who generates a referral. Anything is better than $0 right? Offer a $5 account credit to any existing client who brings in someone that spends $20 or more. If you offer a stellar experience they are more likely to become a lifetime client and you only needed to spend $5 to capture them. That's less than most advertising.

"You can achieve anything you want in life if you have the courage to dream it, the intelligence to make a realistic plan, and the will to see that plan through to the end."
- Sidney A. Friedman

GLOSSARY OF POSES

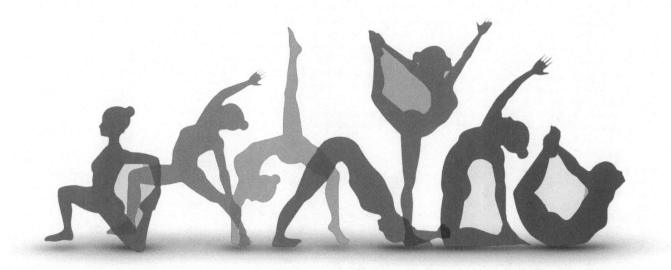

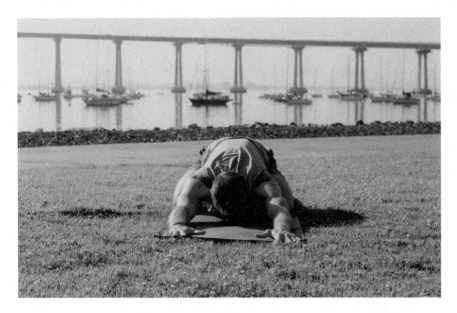

Childs Pose
Balasana

Place a bolster under the chest or hips for support if needed.

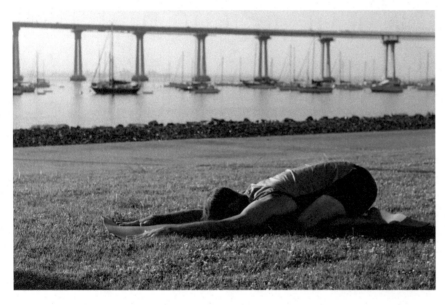

Childs Pose
side view

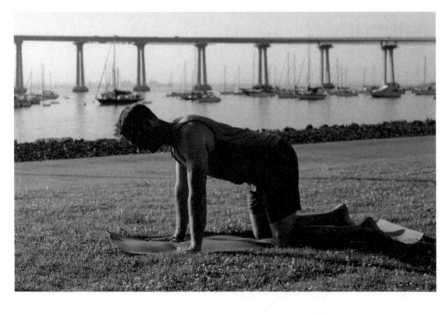

Table Pose
Bharmanasana

200

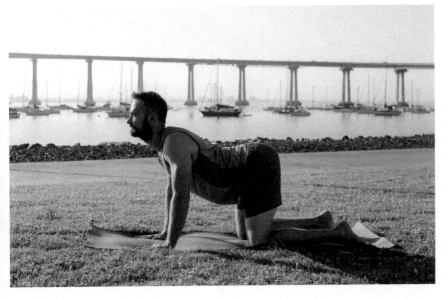

Cat Pose
Marjaryasana

Shoulders over your wrists
& hips over your knees.

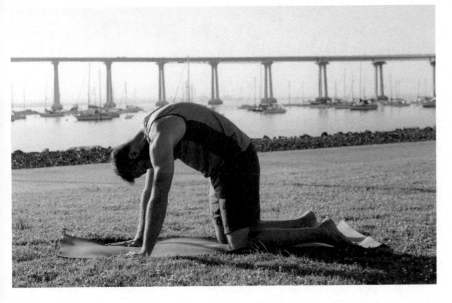

Cow Pose
Bitilasana

Four Limbed Staff
Chaturanga Dandasana

Engage the four inch space
below your bellybutton to
protect your lower back.

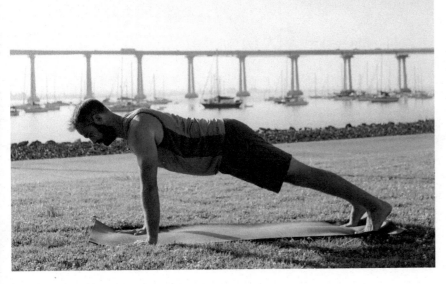

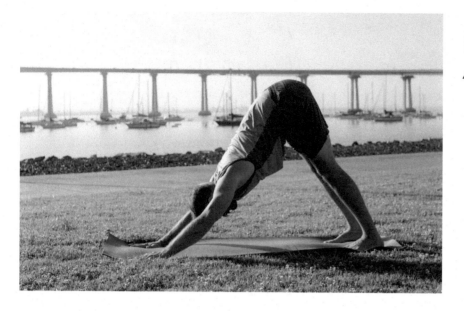

Downdward Dog
Adho Mukha Svanasana

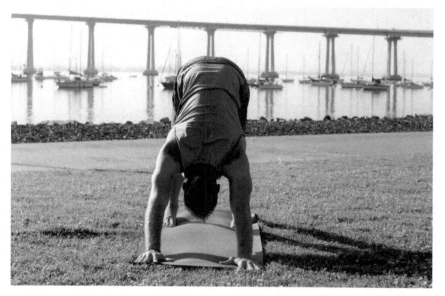

Downward Dog
Front View

Press your hands firmly into the mat engaging your shoulder blades.

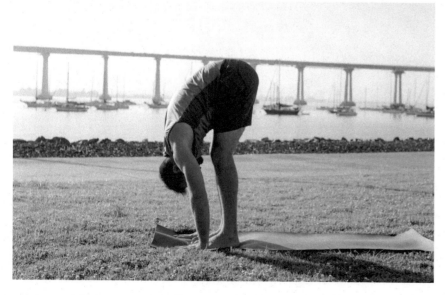

Forward Fold
Uttanasana

Relax your neck, shoulders and back.

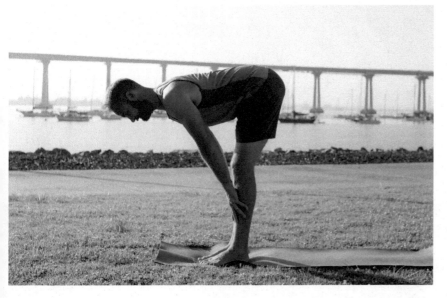

Halfway Lift
Ardha Uttanasana

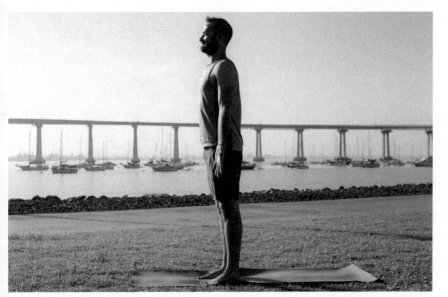

Mountain Pose
Tadasana

Should feel grounded firmly into the earth while still extending towards the heavens.

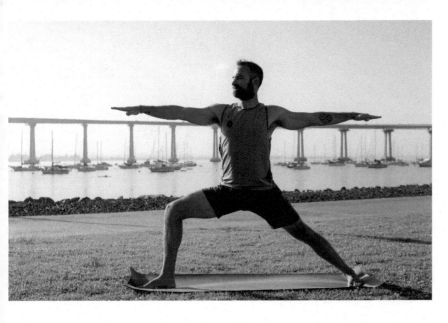

Warrior II
Virabhadrasana II

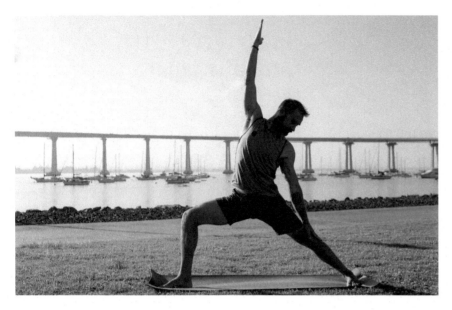

Reverse Warrior
Viparita Virabhadrasana

Try not to put pressure on the back leg with your hand.

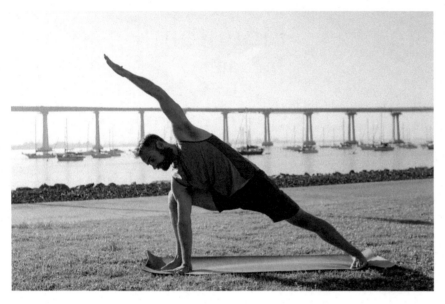

Extended Side Angle
Utthita Parsvakonasana

You can also take the elbow of the bottom arm on top of your knee.

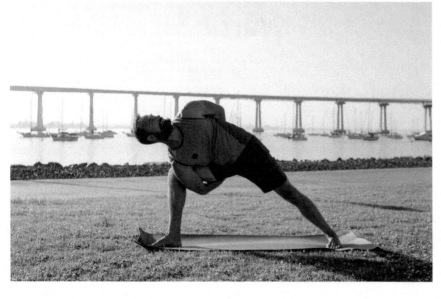

Side Angle Bind
Baddha Parsvakonasana

If a gaze up hurts your neck then look out or down instead.

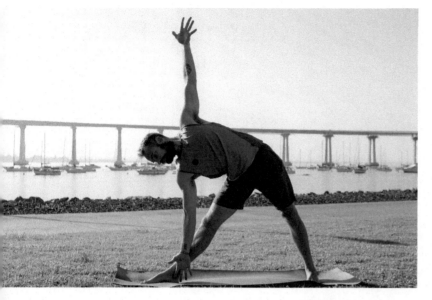

Triangle Pose
Utthita Trikonasana

Press the back of your hand to the medial side of your shin. This engages the upper back and through reciprocal inhibition inhibition opens the chest.

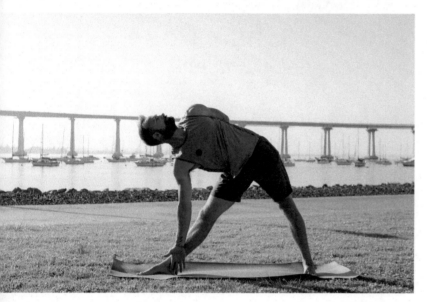

Triangle Bind
Baddha Trikonasana

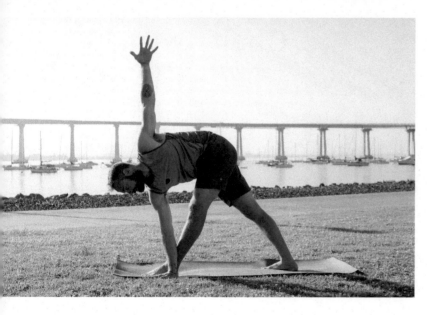

Revolved Triangle
Parivrtta Trikonasana

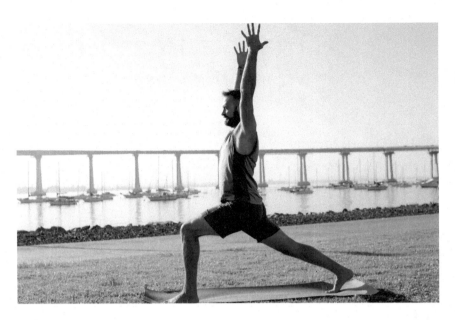

Crescent Pose
Alanasana

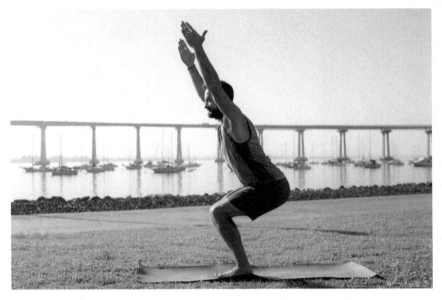

Chair Pose
Utkatasana

Avoid sticking out your tail. There are no "Duck" poses in asana.

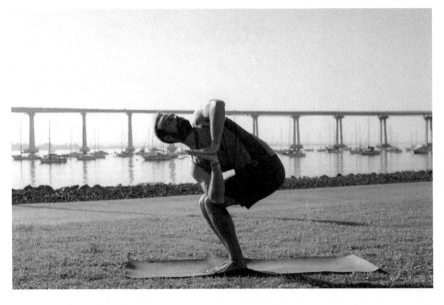

Chair Twist
Parivrtta Utkatasana

It's ok to have one knee out slightly infant of the other.

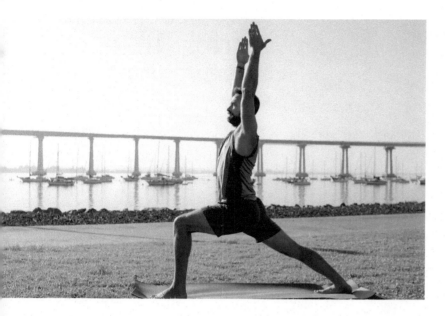

Warrior I
Vihrabhadrasana I

Pyramid Pose
Parsvottanasana

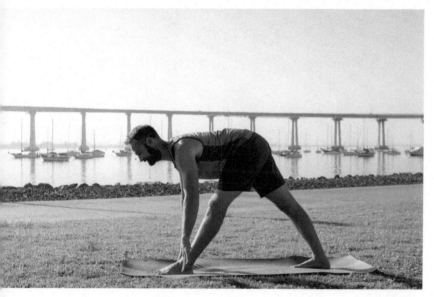

Standing Wide Leg
Prasarita Padottanasana

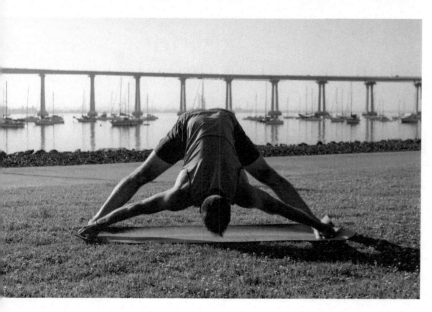

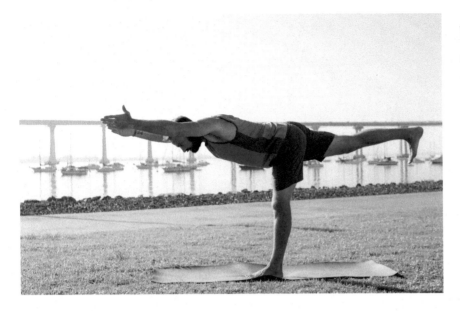

Warrior III
Virabhadrasana III

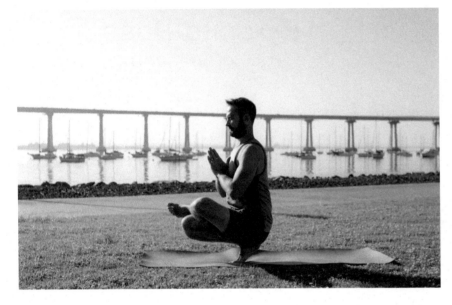

Tiptoe Pose
Pada Angushthasana

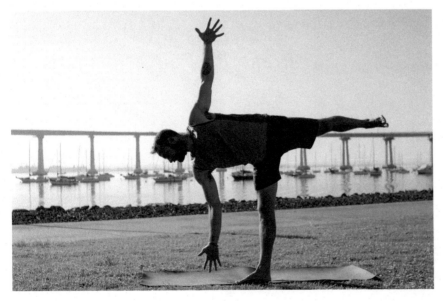

Half Moon Pose
Ardha Chandrasana

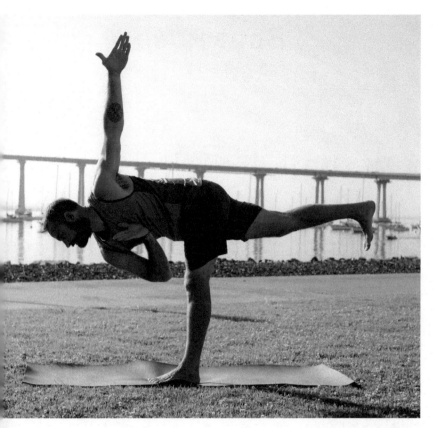

Revolved Half Moon
Parivrtta Ardha Chandrasana

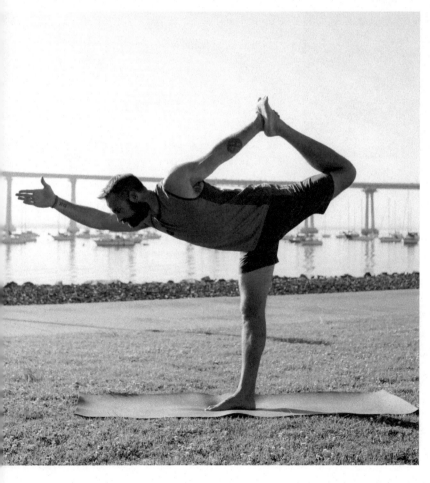

Dancers Pose
Natarajasana

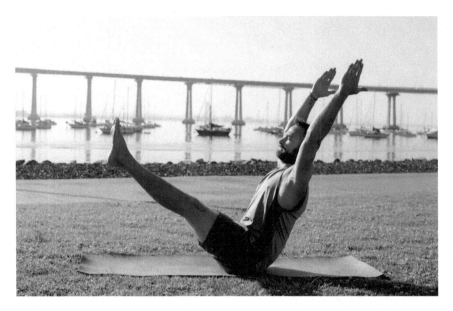

Boat Pose
Navasana

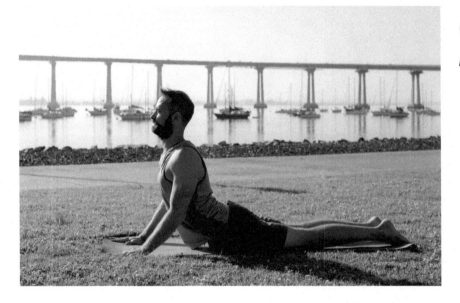

Cobra
Bhujangasana

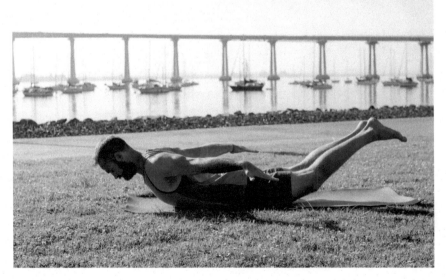

Locust Pose
Salabhasana

Keep your gaze down and your neck neutral.

Bow Pulling Pose
Dhanurasana

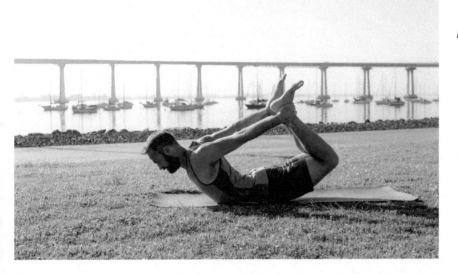

Camel Pose
Ustrasana

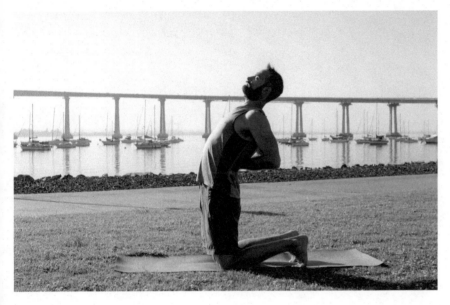

Bridge Pose
Setu Banda Sarvangasana

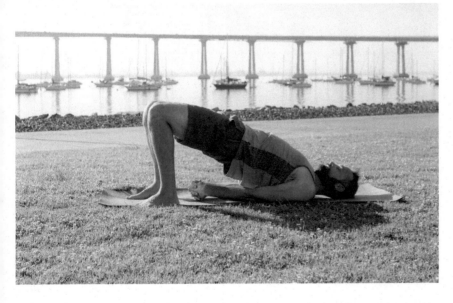

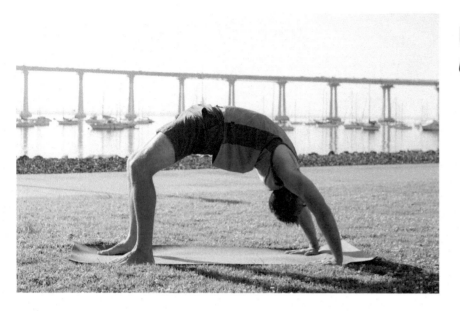

Upward Facing Bow
Urdvha Dhanurasana

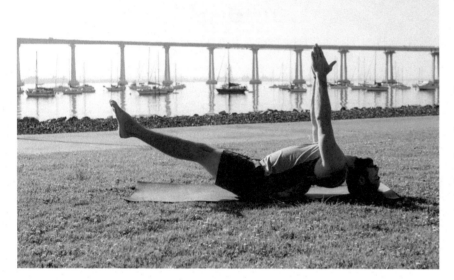

Fish Pose
Matsyasana

The head is here as a point of contact. Avoid placing too much weight to the head, jamming the neck.

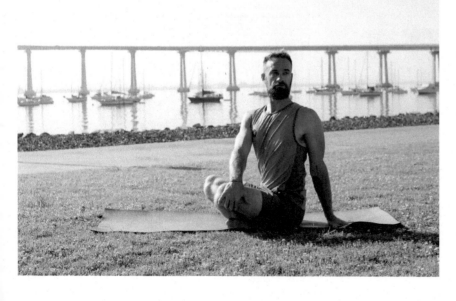

Seated Twist
Parivrtta Sukhasana

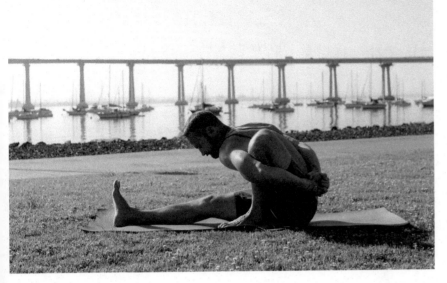

Great Sage Pose I
Marichyasana I

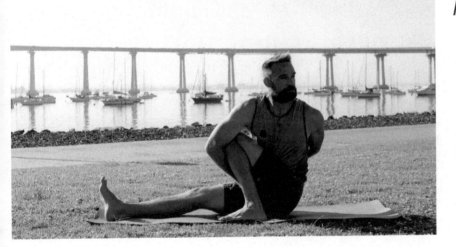

Great Sage Pose II
Marichyasana II

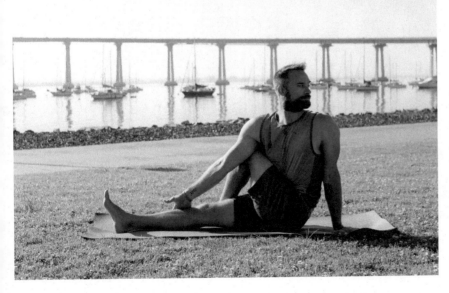

Great Sage Pose II
Marichyasana II

Variation

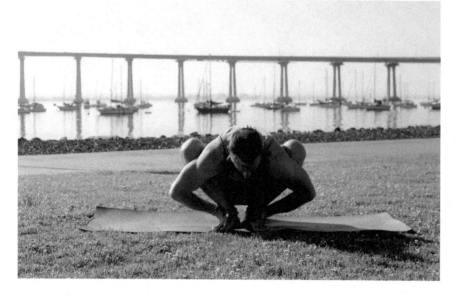

Garland Pose
Malasana

Placing a blanket under your heels in this pose can help with balance.

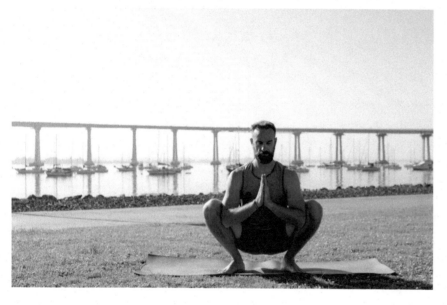

Prayer Squat Pose
Malasana

Place your feet as wide apart as you need to get your heels on the ground.

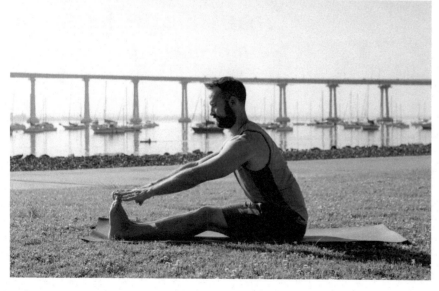

Seated Forward Fold
Paschimottanasana

Option 1 for those with tight hamstrings.

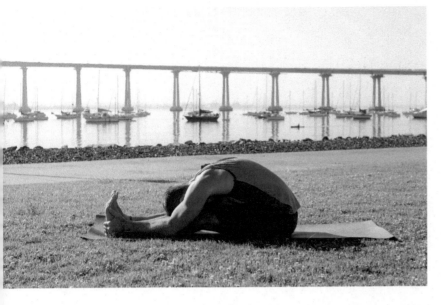

Seated Forward Fold
Paschimottanasana

Option 2 for those with
more flexible hamstrings.

Head-to-Knee
Janu Sirsasana

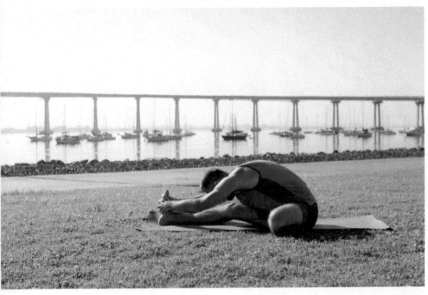

Open Angle Pose
Upavistha Konasana

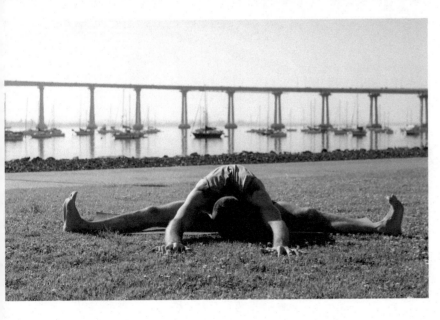

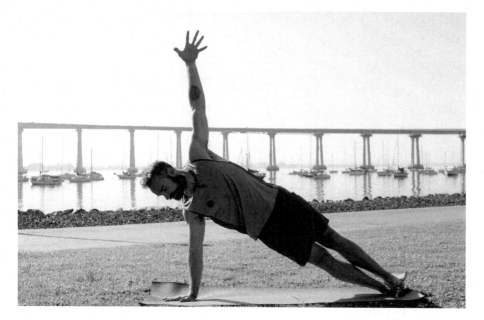

Side Plank
Vasisthasana

Stack your shoulder over your wrist.

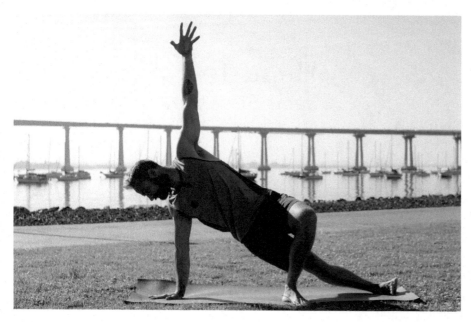

Side Plank
Option

This variation takes some of the pressure off of your arm.

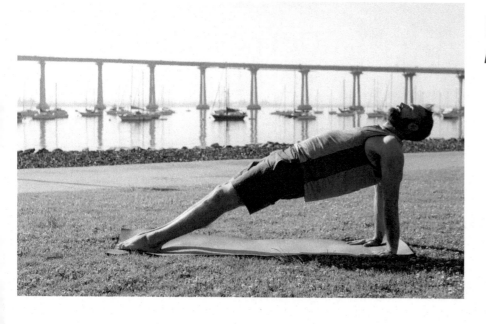

Reverse Plank
Purvottanasana

Crow Pose
Bakasana

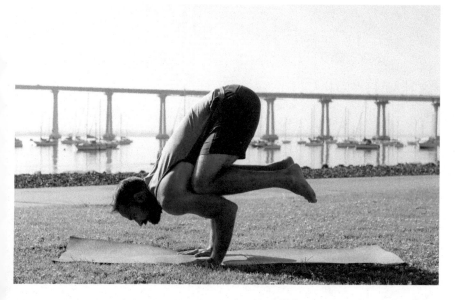

Crane Pose
Bakasana

Variation with arms straight

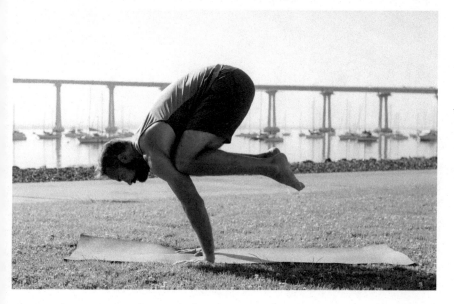

Peacock
Mayurasana

Try not to let your elbows
dig into your belly.

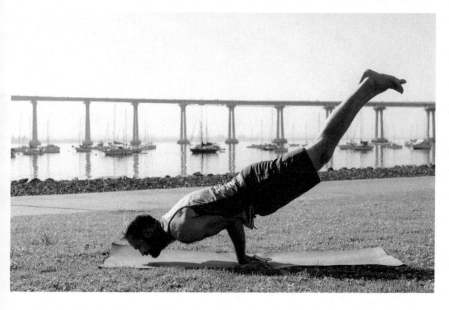

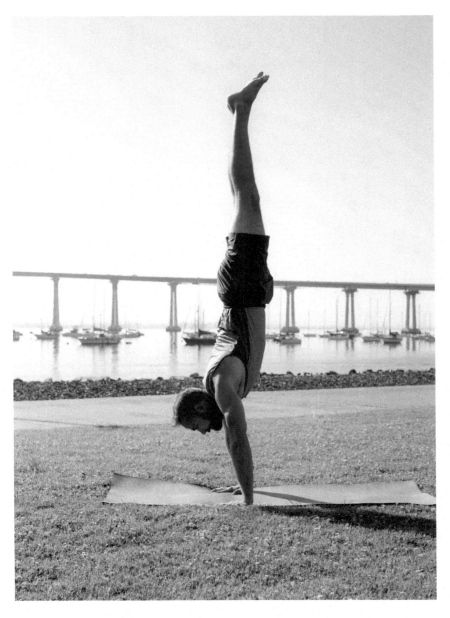

Handstand
Adho Mukha Vrksasana

Press your hands down firmly into the mat, lifting through your feet.

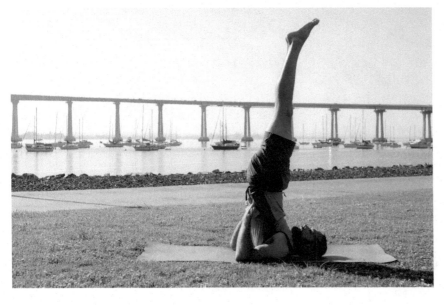

Shoulder Stand
Sarvangasana

Blanket under the shoulders will help keep a neutral position in your cervical spine.

Forearm Stand
Pincha Mayurasana

Avoid a sway in your lower back by tucking your lower ribs and pressing your feet towards the sky.

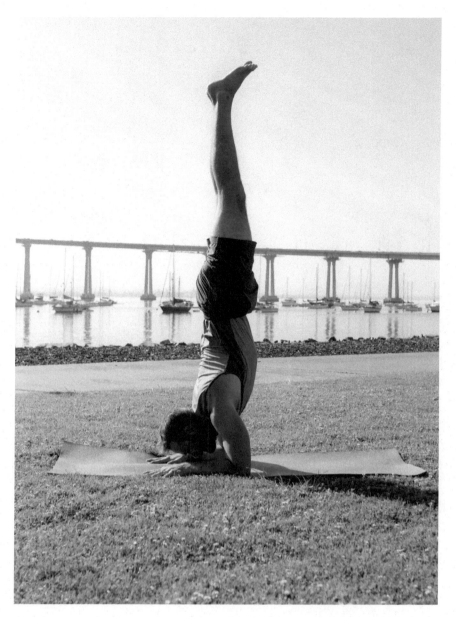

Plow Pose
Halasana

Place a block under the feet if needed.

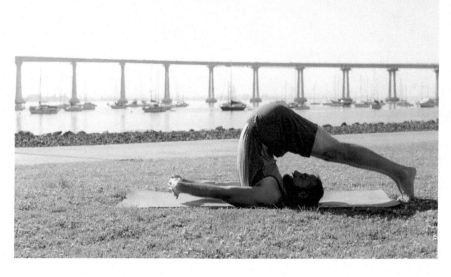

Headstand
Sirsasana

The weight of your body should be dispersed evenly across your arms. Avoid putting all of the weight on your head.

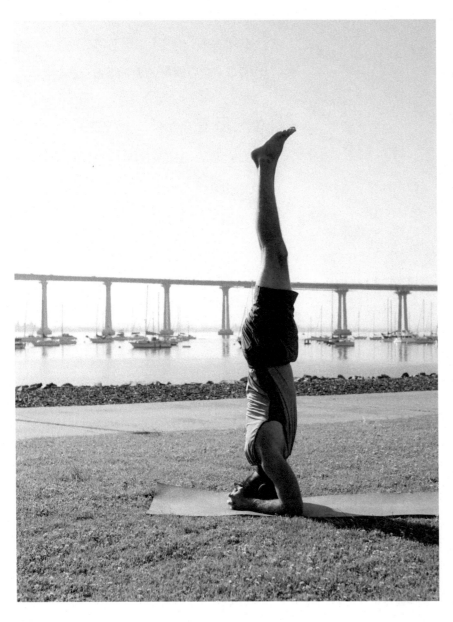

Corpse Pose
Shavasana

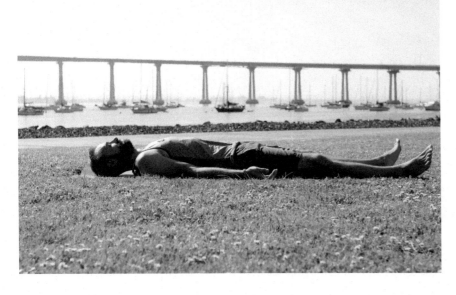

Heros Pose
Virasana

Sit on a block if your knees lift or if there is any pain.

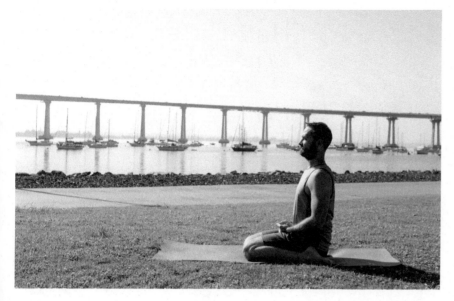

Reclined Heros
Supta Virasana

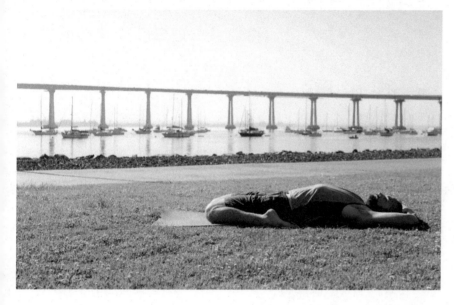

Half Pigeon
Eka Pada Rajakapotasana

Option 1, chest stays lifted.

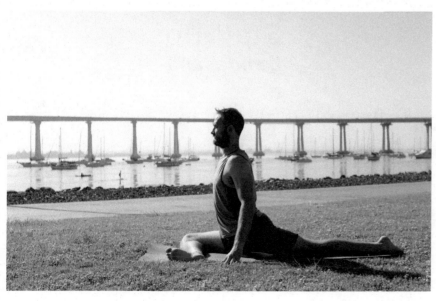

Half Pigeon Pose
Eka Padha Rajakapotasana

Option 2, chest forward and down.

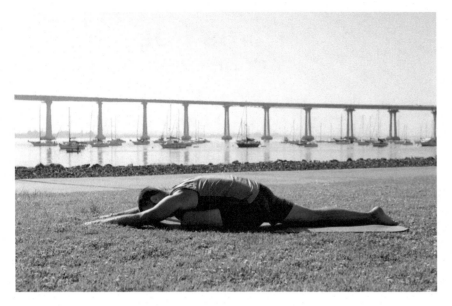

King Pigeon Prep

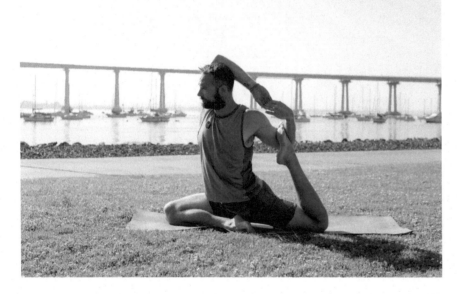

Staff Pose
Dandasana

Tilt your hips forward. Pull your navel in. Press your knees down. Flex your toes back.

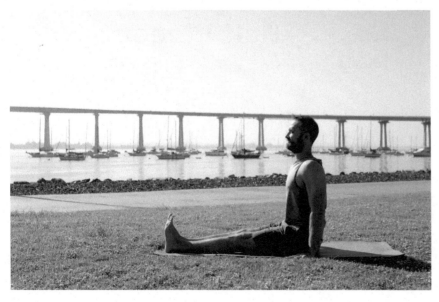

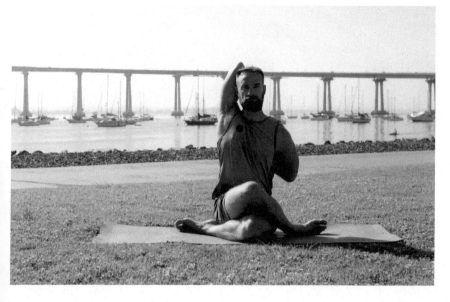

Cow Face Pose
Gomukasana

Use a towel or strap between
the hands if you can't get
the bind.

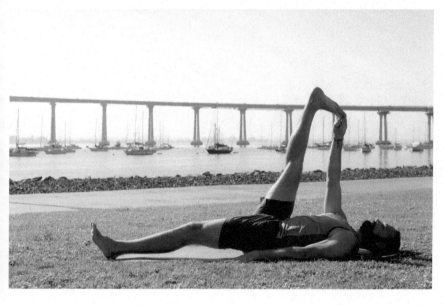

Reclined Big-Toe
Supta Padangusthasana

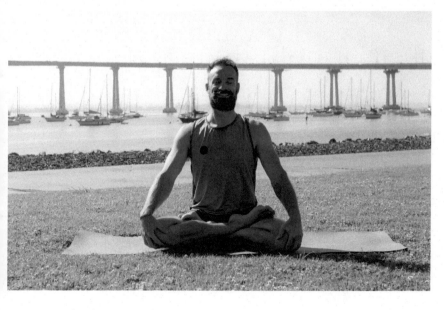

Lotus Pose
Padmasana

Upward Facing Dog
Urdhva Mukha Svanasana

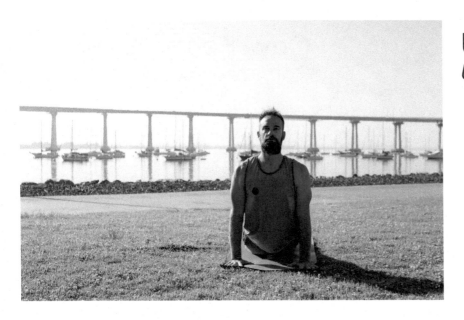

Mountain Pose
Smastitihi

This variation is with the hands together in prayer at heart center.

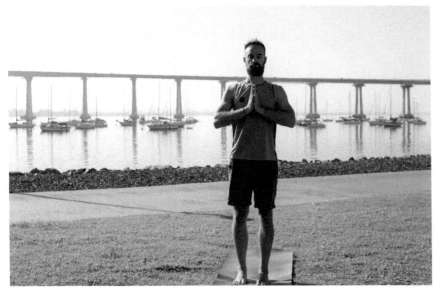

Low Lunge Pose
Anjaneyasana

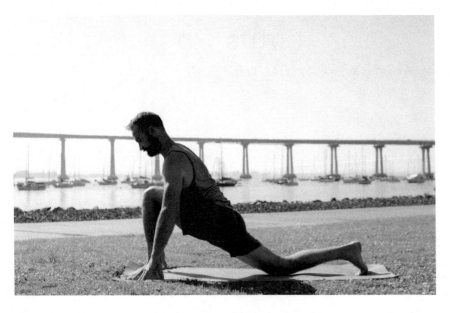

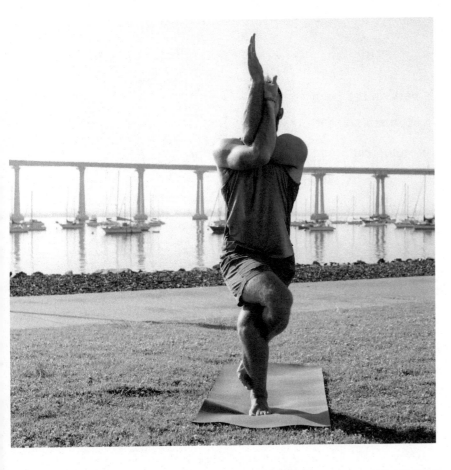

Eagle Pose
Garudasana

Knees and elbows in the same line.

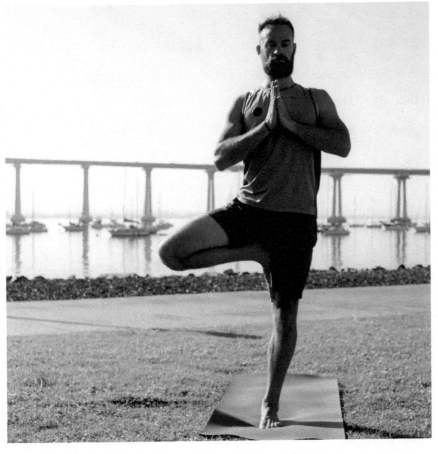

Tree Pose
Vrksasana

You can use a block under the foot of the lifted leg to help with balance.

About the Author

For a majority of his adult life, his passion has been to identify and learn the best services, methods, and philosophies that support and nurture the health and wellness of human beings. In 2005 by the recommendation of his girlfriend (now wife) he was introduced to yoga. It has been a part of his life ever since.

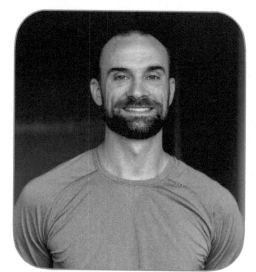

Ryan is a 200-hour Experienced Registered Yoga Teacher (E-RYT) through Yoga Alliance and a member of the International Association of Yoga Therapists. He is the team lead for MOSAIC's Yoga services and the creator and director of their 5-star Yoga Alliance ranked teacher training program.

In 2010, along with my wife and a close friend, he opened his own yoga studio in San Diego California. Ryan currently lives with his wife and three kids in the mountains about 35-minutes outside of downtown San Diego.

Ryan has studied at the National Academy of Sports Medicine, the CHEK Institute for advanced performance, the Metabolic Typing Education Center and Symmetry's school for alignment therapy. He has come to recognize health as the balance and synergy of the human body's many systems, reflected in the way we eat, move, breath, think, rest and surrender.

Ryan has taught over 20,000 students and over 2,000 classes including special operations forces, corporate teams, open enrollment, and professional athletes. He has also trained over 200 yoga teachers. He is a regular headlining teacher at the San Diego Yoga Festival and a contributor to Yoga Digest Magazine.

IG: @RyanLeeGlidden

Email: glidden@exploremosaic.com

Works Cited

American Psychiatric Association. (2013). Diagnostic and statistical manual of mental disorders.

Anderson, C. (2016). *TED TALKS: The Official TED Guide to Public Speaking*. Boston, MA: Hougton Mifflin Harcourt.

Broad, W. J. (2012). *The Science of YOGA: The Risks and the Rewards*. New York, New York: Simon & Schuster.

Brooke Boon, D. D. (2006). *Hatha Yoga Illustrated for Greater Strength, Flexibility, and Focus*. (J. Rhoda, Ed.) Human Kinetics.

Brunson, R. (2017). *Expert Secrets*. New York: Morgan James Publishing.

Carroll, C. a. (2013). *Mudras of India: A Comprehensive Guide to the Hand Gestures of Yoga and Indian Dance*. London, England: Singing Dragon.

Charney, S. M. (2018). *Resilience: The Science of Mastering LIfe's greatest Challenges*. New York, New York: Cambridge University Press.

Chek, P. (2011). *Primal Pattern Movements*. (P. Crozier, Ed.) Vista, CA: C.H.E.K Institute.

Coulter, H. D. (2001). *Anatomy of Hatha Yoga: A Manual for Students, Teachers and Practitioners*. Albany , CA: Body & Breath Inc.

Dale, C. (2009). *The Subtle Body: An encyclopedia of Your Energetic Anatomy*. Boulder, CO: Sounds True, Inc.

David Emerson, E.-R. R. (2009). Trauma-Sensitive Yoga: Principles, Practice, and Research. *International Journal of Yoga Therapy*(19).

Department of Psychology, Yale University. (2013, April). Rethinking stress: the role of mindsets in determining the stress response. *Journal of Personality and Social Psychology*.

Desikachar, T. (1999). *The Heart of Yoga, Developing A Personal Practice*. Rochester, VT: Inner Traditions International.

Desikachar, T. (1999). *The Heart of Yoga: Developing A Personal Practice*. Rochester , Vermont: Inner Traditions International.

Dib, A. (2016). *The 1-Page Marketing Plan: Get New Customers, Make More Money, And Stand Out From The Crowd*. Middletwon, DE, USA: Successwise.

Duhigg, C. (2012). *The Power of Habit: Why We Do What We Do in Life and Business.* New York, New York: Random House.

Feuerstein, G. (1989). *Teh Yoga-Sutra of Patanjali: A New Translation and Commentary.* Rochester, VT: Inner Traditions International.

Feuerstein, G. P. (2009). *Yoga Philosophy and History: An Essential Manual for Yoga Teacher Trainings.* Eastend: Traditional Yoga Studies.

Godin, S. (2008). *TRIBES.* New York: The Penguin Group.

Hartley, L. (1995). *Wisdom of the Body Moving: An Introduction to Body-Mind Centering.* Berkeley: North Atlantic Books.

Iyengar, B. (2005). *Light On Life: The Yoga Journey to Wholeness, Inner Peace, & Ulitmate Freedom.* USA: Rodale Inc.

Iyengar, B. (2008). *YOGA The Path to Holistic Health.* New York, New York: DK Publishing.

Judith, A. (2004). *Eastern Body Western Mind.* New York: Celestial Arts.

Keil, D. (2014). *Functional Anatomy of Yoga.* Chichester: Lotus Publishing.

Keil, K. (2014). *Funtional Anatomy of Yoga a Guide for Practitioners and Teachers.* Chichester, England: Lotus Publishing.

Kolk, B. A. (2002). Beyond the talking cure: somatic experience and subcortical imprints in the treatment of trauma. (F. Shapiro, Ed.) *American Psychological Association,* 57-83.

Kyla Pearce, M. (2016). *Love Your Brain Teacher Training Manual.* training manual, Love Your Brain Foundation.

Lasater, J. H. (2015). Anatomy 101: Understanding Your Sacroiliac Joint. *Yoga Journal.*

Levitin, D. J. (2006). *This Is Your Brain on Music, The Science of a Human Obsession.* New York, New York: Penguin Group.

Long MD, FRCSC, R. (2006). *The Key Muscles of Yoga.* Bandha Yoga Publications.

Marshall Hagins, W. M. (2007). Does practicing hatha yoga satisfy recommendations for intensity of physical activity which improves and maintains health and cardiovascular fitness? *BMC complementary and Alternative Medicine,* 1.

Mathew Thorp, M. P. (2017, July 5). *12 Science-Based Benefits of Meditation*. Retrieved May 19, 2018, from healthline: https://www.healthline.com/nutrition/12-benefits-of-meditation

McGonigal, K. (2015, March 8). *How To Be Good At Stress*. Retrieved March 24, 2018, from IDEAS.TED.COM: https://ideas.ted.com/how-to-be-good-at-stress/

Michael A. Clark, S. C. (Ed.). (2008). *NASM Essentials of Personal Fitness Training* (Third ed.). Baltimore, MD: Lippincott Williams & Wilkins.

Moraitis, a. Y. (2006). *The Healing Power of Your Aura: How to Use Spiritual energy for Physical Heatlh and Well-Being*. Sunland: Spiritual Arts Institute.

Multiple. (2018, January 26th). *Glossophobia*. Retrieved March 18, 2018, from wikipedia.org: https://en.wikipedia.org/wiki/Glossophobia

National Academy of Sports Medicine. (2008). *NASM Essentials of Personal Fitness Training* (3rd ed.). (S. C. Micheal A. Clark, Ed.) Baltimore, MD: Lipincott Williams & Wilkins.

Pat Ogden, k. M. (2006). *Trauma and the Body: A Sensorimotor Approach To Psychotherapy*. New York, New York: W.W. Norton & Company.

Pictures, P. (2010). 3D Anatomy for Yoga: The Essential Guide.

Powers, S. (2008). *Insight Yoga*. Boston: Shambhala Publications.

Ravikanth, B. (2012). *Yoga Sutras of Patanjali: Nature of the mind, the universe, and the true self*. Sanskrit Works.

Richard C. Miller, P. (2015). *The iRest Program for Healing PTSD: A proven-Effective Approach to Using Yoga Nidra Meditation & Deep Relaxation Techniques to Overcome Trauma*. Oakland , California: New Harbinger Publications.

Rick Hanson PH.D. with Richard Mendius, M. (2009). *Buddha's Brain: the practical neuroscience of happiness, love & wisdom*. Oakland, California: New Harbinger Publications, Inc.

Robin, M. (2009). *A Handbook for Yogasana Teachers*. Tucson, AZ: Wheatmark.

Rosen, R. (2006). *Pranayama, Beyond the Fundamentals*. Boston , MA: Shambhala.

Shorter, S. M. (2014). The Vagus Nerves as a Mind-Body Bridge. *Yoga Therapy Today*.

Tosca D. Braun, B. C. (2012). Weight Loss Among Participants in a Residential Kripalu Yoga-Based Weight Loss Program. *International Journal of Yoga Therapy*, 12.

Tosca D. Braun, M. C. (2016). Group-Based Yogic Weight Loss with Ayurveda-Inspired Components: A Pilot Investigation of Female Yoga Practitioners and Novices. *International Journal of Yoga Therapy*.

Vassallo, W. (1990). *Speaking with Confidence: A Guide for Public Speakers*. Crozet, VA: Betterway Publications, Inc.